REAL-WORLD NURSING SURVIVAL GUIDE:
HEMODYNAMIC MONITORING

REAL WORLD ‹NURSING› SURVIVAL GUIDE SERIES

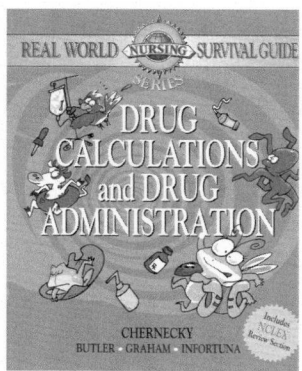

REAL WORLD ‹NURSING› SURVIVAL GUIDE SERIES

DRUG CALCULATIONS and DRUG ADMINISTRATION

Includes NCLEX Review Section

CHERNECKY
BUTLER • GRAHAM • INFORTUNA

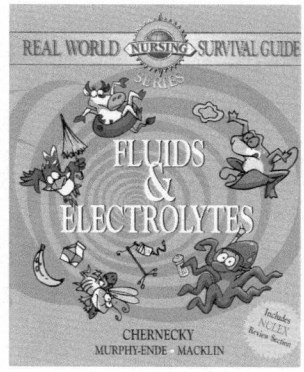

REAL WORLD ‹NURSING› SURVIVAL GUIDE SERIES

FLUIDS & ELECTROLYTES

Includes NCLEX Review Section

CHERNECKY
MURPHY-ENDE • MACKLIN

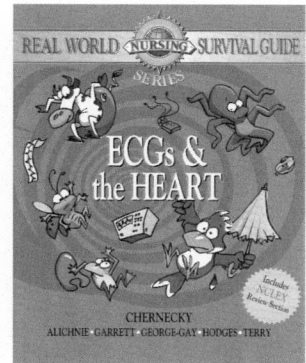

REAL WORLD ‹NURSING› SURVIVAL GUIDE SERIES

ECGs & the HEART

Includes NCLEX Review Section

CHERNECKY
ALICHNIE • GARRETT • GEORGE-GAY • HODGES • TERRY

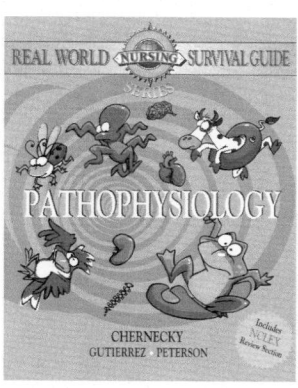

REAL WORLD ‹NURSING› SURVIVAL GUIDE SERIES

PATHOPHYSIOLOGY

Includes NCLEX Review Section

CHERNECKY
GUTIERREZ • PETERSON

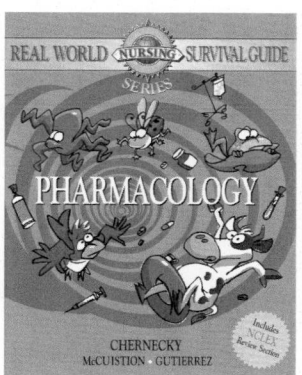

REAL WORLD ‹NURSING› SURVIVAL GUIDE SERIES

PHARMACOLOGY

Includes NCLEX Review Section

CHERNECKY
McCUISTION • GUTIERREZ

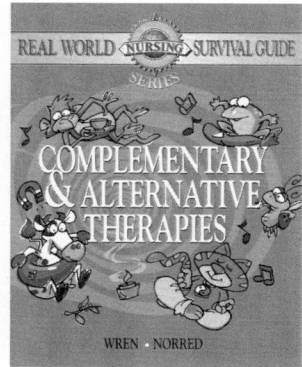

REAL WORLD ‹NURSING› SURVIVAL GUIDE SERIES

COMPLEMENTARY & ALTERNATIVE THERAPIES

WREN • NORRED

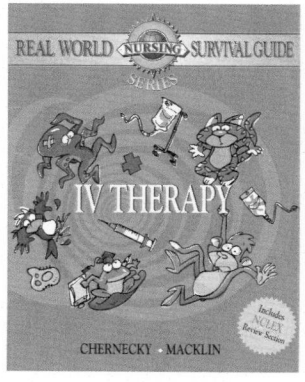

REAL WORLD ‹NURSING› SURVIVAL GUIDE SERIES

IV THERAPY

Includes NCLEX Review Section

CHERNECKY • MACKLIN

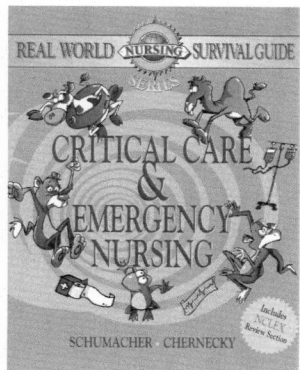

REAL WORLD ‹NURSING› SURVIVAL GUIDE SERIES

CRITICAL CARE & EMERGENCY NURSING

Includes NCLEX Review Section

SCHUMACHER • CHERNECKY

REAL-WORLD NURSING SURVIVAL GUIDE:

HEMODYNAMIC MONITORING

REBECCA K. HODGES, MSN, RN, CCRN
Critical Care Clinical Nurse Specialist
St. Joseph Hospital
Augusta, Georgia

KITTY M. GARRETT, MSN, RN, CCRN
Critical Care Clinical Nurse Specialist
St. Joseph Hospital
Augusta, Georgia

CYNTHIA CHERNECKY, PhD, RN, CNS, AOCN
Professor, Department of Adult Health
Medical College of Georgia, School of Nursing
Augusta, Georgia

LORI SCHUMACHER, PhD, RN, CCRN
Assistant Professor
Medical College of Georgia, School of Nursing
Augusta, Georgia

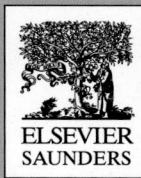

ELSEVIER
SAUNDERS

ELSEVIER
SAUNDERS

11830 Westline Industrial Drive
St. Louis, Missouri 63146

REAL-WORLD NURSING SURVIVAL GUIDE:
HEMODYNAMIC MONITORING

ISBN 978-0-7216-0375-9

NOTICE

Nursing is an ever-changing field. Standard safety precautions must be followed, but as new research and clinical experience broaden our knowledge, changes in treatment and drug therapy may become necessary or appropriate. Readers are advised to check the most current product information provided by the manufacturer of each drug to be administered to verify the recommended dose, the method and duration of administration, and contraindications. It is the responsibility of the licensed prescriber, relying on experience and knowledge of the patient, to determine dosages and the best treatment for each individual patient. Neither the publisher nor the author assumes any liability for any injury and/or damage to persons or property arising from this publication.

International Standard Book Number 978-0-7216-0375-9

Executive Vice President, Nursing and Health Professions: Sally Schrefer
Executive Publisher: Robin Carter
Developmental Editor: Deanna Davis
Publishing Services Manager: Melissa Lastarria
Senior Designer: Amy Buxton
Cover Art: GraphCom Corporation

Printed in the United States of America

Transferred to Digital Printing in 2013

About the Authors

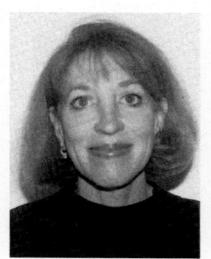

Rebecca (Becki) Hodges earned her MSN and BSN from the Medical College of Georgia. She is a Critical Care Clinical Nurse Specialist at St. Joseph Hospital in Augusta, Georgia, with over 27 years experience in an acute care setting. Becki has maintained CCRN certification for over 20 years and was a charter member and past president of the CSRA chapter of AACN. She was awarded the Leilee P. Ault Clinical Excellence in Graduate Adult Nursing Award from the Medical College of Georgia and has been named to *Who's Who in Nursing*. She has been actively involved in consulting and lecturing and has authored chapters on critical care topics. Becki is an avid gardener, specializing in garden design.

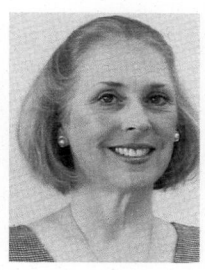

Kitty Garrett earned her MSN and BSN degrees from the Medical College of Georgia. She is a Critical Care Clinical Nurse Specialist at St. Joseph Hospital in Augusta, Georgia. She has 25 years of experience teaching basic dysrhythmias, 12-lead ECGs, and BCLS, ACLS, and CCRN reviews. She is a national and local member of AACN and has maintained CCRN certification for 20 years. She also serves as a part-time clinical faculty member for the School of Nursing at the Medical College of Georgia. Kitty enjoys gardening, walking, playing tennis, and teaching Sunday school classes to teenagers.

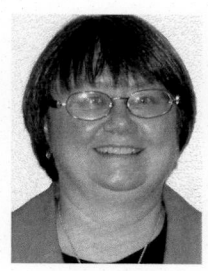

Dr. Cynthia Chernecky earned her degrees at the Case Western Reserve University (PhD), the University of Pittsburgh (MN), and the University of Connecticut (BSN). She also earned an NCI fellowship at Yale University and a postdoctorate visiting scholarship at UCLA. Her clinical area of expertise is critical care oncology with publications including *Laboratory Tests and Diagnostic Procedures* (fourth edition) and *Advanced and Critical Care Oncology Nursing: Managing Primary Complications*. She is a national speaker, researcher, and published scholar in cancer nursing. She is also active in the Orthodox Church and enjoys life with family, friends, colleagues, and two West Highland white terriers.

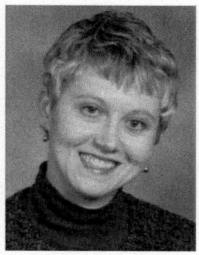

Lori Schumacher earned her degrees at Duquesne University (PhD), Creighton University (BSN), and the University of Minnesota (MS). She has over 15 years of experience in critical care and neuroscience nursing and maintains CCRN certification. She is active in her church and an accomplished flutist. Lori enjoys giving flute lessons and spending time with her family, friends, and four cats.

Contributors

Brenda L. Garman, RN, BSN, MED
Education Specialist, Learning Resources
St. Joseph Hospital
Augusta, Georgia

Richard Hass, PhD, CRNA
Assistant Professor, Nursing Anesthesia Program
Medical College of Georgia
Augusta, Georgia

Lee Dorman, MN, CRNA

Faculty and Student Reviewers

FACULTY

Mamoona Arif, MSN
Critical Care Clinical Nurse Specialist
Manassas Park, Virginia

Jennifer Kane, RN, BSN

Patricia A. Knowles, RN, CCRN
John Freeman Intensive Care Unit
Addenbrookes Hospital
Cambridge
Cambridgeshire, England

Kara A. Lauze, NP
Acute Care Nurse Practitioner
Critical Care Unit
University of Massachusetts Medical
  Center
Worcester, Massachusetts

Theresa Posani, PhD(c), RN, CNS, CS,
  CCNS, CCRN
Lecturer, Nursing Department
Louise Herrington School of Nursing
Baylor University
Dallas, Texas

Marilyn (Mimi) Rose, MSN, RN, CCRN
Clinical Nurse Specialist, Critical
  Care
Enloe Medical Center
Chico, California

Joy Speciale, RN, MBA, CCRN
Assistant Director of Cardiology
CVICU, CCU, and Intermediate Care
Hinsdale Hospital
Hinsdale, Illinois

Laurel Tyler, RN, MN, CCRN
Department of Critical Care
University of Washington
Seattle, Washington

Gail Vitale, MS, APRN, BC
Assistant Professor
College of Nursing and Health
  Professions
Lewis University
Romeoville, Illinois

Jackie Yon, RN, MS, CCRN, CCNS
Director of Cardiac Services
Cardiac Specialty Care Center
Lakeland Regional Medical Center
Lakeland, Florida

STUDENTS

The following students from Saint Louis University, School of Nursing, St. Louis, Missouri, helped the editors shape the vision of this reference through focus group reviews and breakout sessions:

Megan A. Kellon, BSN
Casey Elizabeth McCoy, RN, BSN
Michelle Monteilh, RN, BSN

Sreeja Manchira Natesan
Kathryn Parker, RN, BSN
Julie A Podlogar, RN, BSN

Gina B. Scully, BSN
Melanie S. Szymanski, RN, BSN

Preface

The Real-World Nursing Survival Guide series was created with your input. Nursing students told us about topics they found difficult to master, such as hemodynamics and critical care and emergency. Based on information from focus groups at the National Student Nurses Association meeting, this series was developed on your recommendations. You said to keep the text to a minimum; to use an engaging, fun approach; to provide enough space to write on the pages; to include a variety of activities to appeal to the different learning styles of students; to make the content visually appealing; and to provide NCLEX review questions so you could check your understanding of key topics and review as necessary. This series is a result of your ideas!

Understanding the concepts and principles of hemodynamic monitoring provides a solid foundation for the nurse working with critically ill patients to guide drug therapy, monitor hemodynamic parameters, and make sound clinical decisions for nursing interventions. It is essential for any nurse working in critical care to be aware of the importance and use of this technology. Comprehension of this complex maze of equipment, waveforms, alarms, and digital readouts can be overwhelming.

Hemodynamic Monitoring in the *Real World Nursing Survival Guide* series was developed to explain difficult concepts in an easy-to-understand manner and to assist nursing students in the mastery of these concepts. This book can also serve as a valuable guide for experienced nurses and clinicians who want to review the principles of hemodynamic monitoring.

We include many features in the margins to help you focus on the vital information you will need to succeed in the classroom and in the clinical setting. **TAKE HOME POINTS** are composed of both study tips for classroom tests and "pearls of wisdom" to assist you in caring for patients. Both are drawn from our many years of combined academic and clinical experience. Content marked with a **Caution** icon is vital and usually involves nursing actions that may have life-threatening consequences or may significantly affect patient outcomes. The **Lifespan** icon 🐢 and the **Culture** icon 🌓 highlight variations in treatment that may be necessary for specific age or ethnic groups. A **Calculator** icon 🖩 will draw your eye to important formulas. A **Web Links** icon 🖥 will direct you to sites on the Internet that will give more detailed information on a given topic. Each of these icons is designed to help you focus on real-world patient care, the nursing process, and positive patient outcomes.

We also use consistent headings that emphasize specific nursing actions. **What It IS** provides a definition of a topic. **What You NEED TO KNOW** provides the explanation of the topic. **What You DO** explains what you do as a practicing nurse. **Patient Education Points** are marked with a special bullet in this section. **Do You UNDERSTAND?** provides questions and exercises that are both entertaining and useful to reinforce the topic's concepts. This four-step approach provides you with information and helps you learn how to apply it to the clinical setting.

Our goal is for this book to make a difficult topic easier. We have used real-world clinical experiences and expertise to bring you a text that will help you understand hemodynamic monitoring and facilitate better patient care. The art and science of nursing is based on understanding, which is the key to critical thinking. Share your new insights and understanding with others, and apply this information to affect nursing care positively.

Rebecca K. Hodges, MSN, RN, CCRN
Kitty M. Garrett, MSN, RN, CCRN
Cynthia C. Chernecky, PhD, RN, CNS, AOCN
Lori Schumacher, PhD, RN, CCRN

Acknowledgments

To my husband and best friend, Jack, and my son Stuart, who provide me with unfailing love and support. I can never thank you enough! My life is so very blessed with special friends, family, and colleagues who continue to make life a joy. To my mother, sisters, and brothers, our journey has been blessed. A special thank you to the ICU staff and to my colleagues at St. Joseph Hospital and to my friend, co-editor, and partner, Kitty Garrett, who is always there with support.

This book would not be a reality without the persuasion of Dr. Cinda Chernecky, my mentor and friend. In memory of the special people who have touched my life: my dad, Dr. Hubert King, my lifelong friend, Almer, and Dr. Hurley Jones. Thanks also to Dr. Wade Strickland who, along with Dr. Jones, introduced me to the joys of cardiology. Finally, thank you to Paige, Brad, Havird, Hodges, Phyllis, Rob, Riah, Tamara, Blake, and Jordan who always love me back, and to my friend, Lynn Cody, who always keeps life in the proper perspective.

Becki Hodges

Hemodynamics is not an easy topic to understand. As a critical care nurse, I struggled with it for several years before I finally understood it. I am happy to have an opportunity to share some of the ideas that have helped me through the years. I have had many mentors. I would like to thank Maurene Harvey whose CCRN Review first helped it all make sense. Thank you to all of the cardiologists—Dr. Harry Harper, Dr. John Kelly, Dr. Paul Cundey, Dr. Scott Key, Dr. Abdulla Abdulla, and Dr. Mac Bowman—for numerous talks on preload, afterload, and contractility, and their relationships to drugs and interventions. I would like to thank Dr. Cynthia Chernecky for her infinite wisdom and her "gentle" persuasion that this book should be written. This dream would not have become a reality without her guidance. Where would I be without my friend, partner, and co-editor, Becki Hodges? We have struggled through learning creative ways to teach hemodynamic concepts together for the past 15 years. Finally, I certainly could not have contributed my time and energy into this endeavor without the patience and support of my husband, Mike, and my children, Trey, Brian, and Michael, my daughters-in-law, Kelly and Lori, and my grand-daughters, Ansley and Mary Lorick, who remind me when it is time to take a break.

Kitty Garrett

This book is an excellent example of the power within nursing as a practice and a discipline. The editors and authors are clinical experts. They used their collective knowledge and incorporated the areas of research and education to produce outcomes that are relevant to each and every student and practicing nurse. Without the support and respect of each other, this book would never have been accomplished. You will find no better professionals than the individuals associated with this text; we know in our hearts that our working together will make a difference for many in health care. I am very lucky to have met and worked with such wonderful people as Becki, Kitty, Lori, and all the others associated with this project. I also want to acknowledge those that serve as my mentors, who know a lot about excellence, perseverance, and dedication: Dr. Ann Kolanowski, Dr. Linda Sarna, Dr. Jean Brown, Dr. Mary Cooley, and Dr. G. Padilla. Finally, there are several people who support me and make my daily life truly a joy; my mother Olga, my Godmother Helen, and the nuns (Abbess Thecla, Mother Helena, Mother Seraphima) of Saints Mary and Martha Orthodox Monastery in South Carolina.

Cynthia (Cinda) Chernecky

I would like to thank my family, colleagues, and students who have supported and encouraged me during the process of making this book a reality. To my father and mother, Stan and Sandy, who have inspired me in all my nursing endeavors. I also thank all the critical care nurses at Buffalo General Hospital for their diligence and care that they rendered to my father during his numerous visits to their ICUs—without you, great things would not be possible! I would also like to express a special thanks to the doctoral faculty at Duquesne University, especially Dr. Joannie Lockhart and Dr. Gladys Husted, for their inspiration and encouragement through my doctoral studies and the publishing of this book. Finally, I would like to thank my mentor and colleague, Cinda Chernecky, for her patience, confidence, and willingness to nurture me through this process.

Lori Schumacher

Contents

1 Understanding the Heart & Lungs

Hemodynamic monitoring allows for the measurement of pressures in the circulatory system, heart, and lungs. Because the circulatory, cardiovascular, and pulmonary systems are so closely interrelated, the health care provider must understand the anatomy, physiology, and relationship of these systems to comprehend fully how to measure hemodynamic pressures.

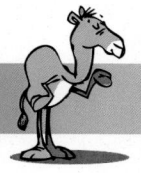

What IS the Anatomy and Physiology of the Circulatory System and the Heart?

The body has a complex network of veins and arteries in a continuous circuit that make up the circulatory system. The heart pumps a constant volume of blood through this system to maintain balance between oxygen delivery and demand. The circulatory system, heart, and conduction system must work together for the heart to beat efficiently (see Color Plates 1 and 2).

The heart is a muscular organ about the size of an adult's clenched fist. The function of the heart is to pump blood through the vascular system to the tissues to meet the metabolic demands of the body. The heart has three main layers: the *endocardium* (the inner layer), the *myocardium* (the main, muscular layer), and the *epicardium* (the outer layer). Another layer, called the *pericardium*, is a dense fibrous outer sac that acts as a cushion to protect the heart.

The heart is made up of two upper chambers called the *atria* and two lower chambers called the *ventricles*. The atria serve as reservoirs for incoming blood, and the ventricles are the main pumping chambers of the heart. The

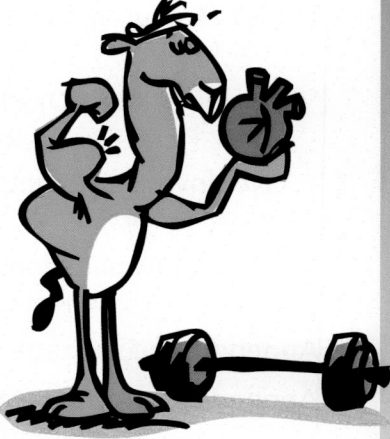

1

atria are separated from the ventricles by atrioventricular valves (AV valves). The tricuspid valve separates the right atrium from the right ventricle and the mitral valve separates the left atrium from the left ventricle. Two other valves, the pulmonic and aortic, help control the flow of blood from the ventricles to the lungs and systemic circulation. The pulmonic semilunar valve controls the flow of blood from the right ventricle to the lungs, and the aortic semilunar valve controls the flow of blood from the left ventricle to the aorta. The septum separates the right side of the heart from the left side of the heart.

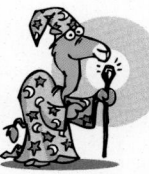 # What You NEED TO KNOW

The heart functions as two different pumps. The right heart pumps desaturated blood to the lungs to drop off carbon dioxide and pick up oxygen. The left heart pumps oxygenated blood to the tissues. Under normal circumstances the pressure in the lungs is low and the pressure in the aorta and systemic circulation is much higher. Therefore the left ventricle is thicker in muscle mass and generates higher pressures than the right ventricle.

Both sides of the heart work together. While the right ventricle is ejecting blood to the pulmonary artery and to the lungs, the left ventricle is ejecting blood to the aorta (see Color Plate 3).

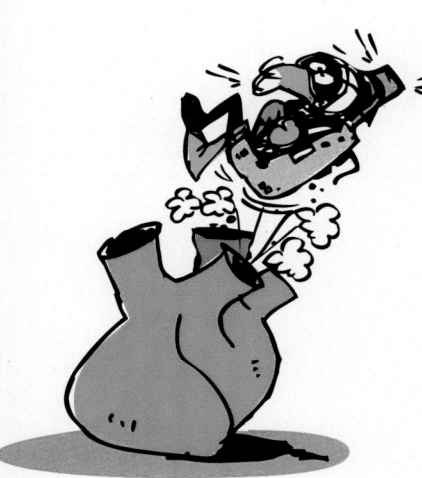

The right atrium receives venous blood from the inferior and superior vena cava. Blood travels from the right atrium through the tricuspid valve to the right ventricle. It is then ejected from the right ventricle through the pulmonic valve to the pulmonary artery and pulmonary capillary bed. At this point an exchange of oxygen and carbon dioxide occur.

Oxygenated blood returns to the left atrium through four pulmonary veins—two from the right lung and two from the left lung. The pulmonary veins do not contain any valves. Blood flows from the left atrium to the left ventricle through the mitral valve. Blood is ejected from the left ventricle through the aortic valve to the aorta and systemic circulation.

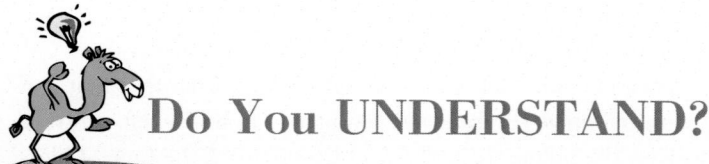

Do You UNDERSTAND?

DIRECTIONS: **Fill in the blanks to complete the following statements.**

1. The function of the heart is to _____

   blood through the vascular system.

2. The upper chambers of the heart are called _____,

   and the lower chambers are _____.

3. The main, muscular layer of the heart is called the

   _____.

4. The right side of the heart pumps desaturated blood to the

   _____ to drop off carbon dioxide and pick up oxygen.

5. Oxygenated blood returns to the left atrium by way of _____

   _____.

6. The pulmonary veins have _____ valves.

DIRECTIONS: **Match each statement in Column A with its answer in Column B.**

Column A	Column B
_____ 7. This valve separates the right atrium from the right ventricle.	a. AV
_____ 8. This valve separates the right ventricle from the pulmonary artery.	b. mitral
_____ 9. This valve separates the left atrium from the left ventricle.	c. pulmonic
_____ 10. The atria are separated from the ventricles by these valves.	d. tricuspid

Answers: 1. pump; 2. atria, ventricles; 3. myocardium; 4. lungs; 5. four pulmonary veins; 6. no; 7. d; 8. c; 9. b; 10. a.

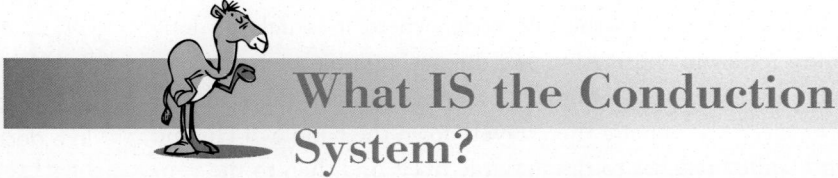

What IS the Conduction System?

The electrical conduction system is specialized tissue that allows electrical impulses to travel efficiently from the atria to the ventricles. This system is composed of the sinoatrial node (SA node), internodal tracts, atrioventricular node (AV node), bundle of His, right and left bundle branches, Purkinje fibers, and ventricular cells.

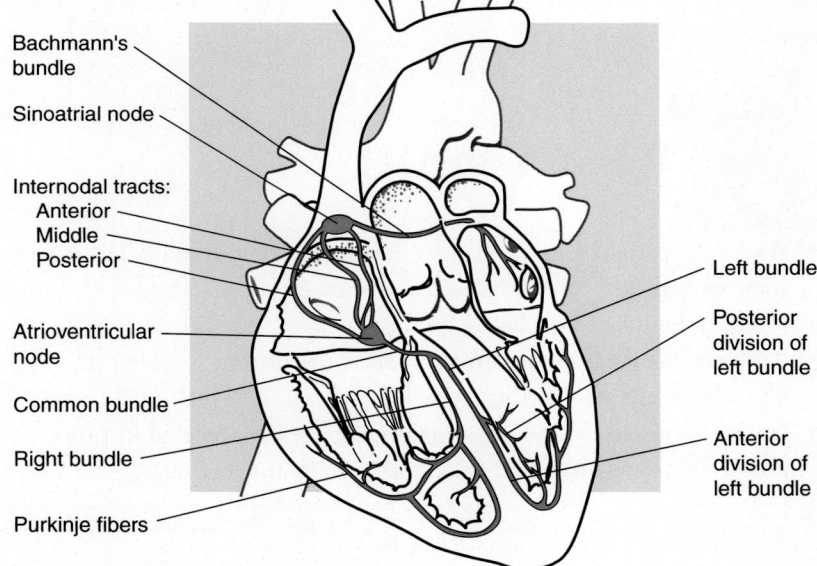

Bachmann's bundle

Sinoatrial node

Internodal tracts:
  Anterior
  Middle
  Posterior

Atrioventricular node

Common bundle

Right bundle

Purkinje fibers

Left bundle

Posterior division of left bundle

Anterior division of left bundle

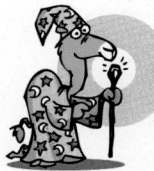

What You NEED TO KNOW

The SA node acts as the pacemaker of the heart and has the ability to fire and recover 60 to 100 times per minute. It consists of a bundle of nerve fibers located at the junction of the superior vena cava and right atrium. The impulse from the SA node travels through the atrium and depolarizes atrial cells. *Depolarization* is the electrical activation of the muscle cells of the heart. This electrical activation is the stimulation for cellular contraction.

The electrical impulse reaches the AV node, where it is delayed long enough to allow for atrial contraction and the optimization of ventricular filling. This action promotes coordinated pumping between the atria and ventricles. The electrical impulse then travels down the bundle of His and right and left bundle branches to the Purkinje fibers and then to the ventricular cells, causing ventricular depolarization. Cellular contraction follows the depolarization process. Once the cells of the heart are depolarized, the cells return to their original state of electrolyte balance, which is called *repolarization*.

The impulses that travel through the conduction system to depolarize the heart can be recorded on an electrocardiogram (ECG). On the ECG, one cardiac cycle is represented by waveforms, which can be analyzed and measured.

- Aging increases the thickness of the left ventricle.
- Increased age results in a decrease in maximal heart rate with exercise, reducing maximal performance.
- Aging **does not affect** cardiac output, but the heart pumps less efficiently as age advances.

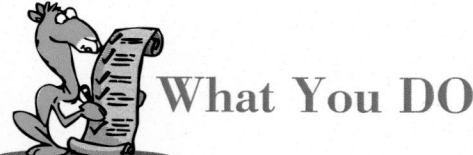

What You DO

- Assess the patient for any changes in heart rate and rhythm. Heart rates that are too fast (tachycardias), too slow (bradycardias), or irregular result in diminished cardiac output.
- Note any medications or herbal products the patient is taking that may affect heart rate and rhythm.
- Follow advanced cardiac life support guidelines or accepted institutional protocols for any change in rhythm that is life threatening.

For further information on advanced cardiac life support, visit www.Americanheart.org.

SIGNS AND SYMPTOMS OF DIMINISHED CARDIAC OUTPUT

- Hypotension (orthostatic hypotension may indicate hypovolemia)
- Increased capillary refill time (greater than 3 seconds)
- Changes in level of consciousness (LOC)
- Decreased urinary output
- Changes in pulse rate
- Other signs of poor perfusion (e.g., chest pain, shortness of breath)

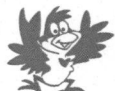

For further information on the electrical conduction system and ECG interpretation, see the *Real World Nursing Survival Guide: ECGs & the Heart* at http://www.us.elsevierhealth.com/product.jsp?isbn=072169036X.

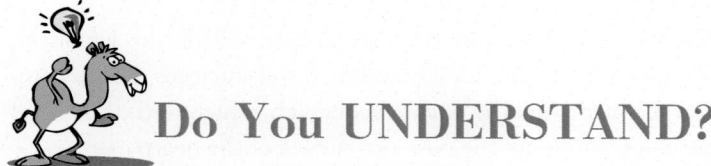

Do You UNDERSTAND?

DIRECTIONS: **Select the correct answer from those provided within the parentheses.**

1. The _____ _____

   system provides electrical activation to cause the heart to pump.

   (*cardiac conduction, coronary artery*)

2. The _____ _____ is considered

   the main pacemaker of the heart. (*SA node, AV node*)

3. Aging _____ the thickness of the

   left ventricle. (*decreases, increases*)

4. Cellular contraction follows the process of _____.

   (*repolarization, depolarization*)

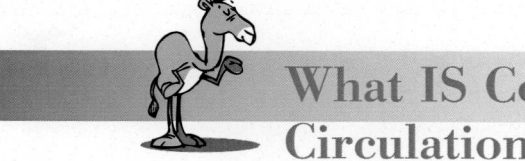

What IS Coronary Circulation?

Vascular changes with aging include the following:
* Arteries lose their elasticity.
* Arterial walls thicken and harden.

The blood supply to the heart muscle (myocardium) is provided through the coronary arteries.

1. The right coronary artery and its branches, which feed the right ventricle (In the majority of individuals, it feeds the SA node, AV node, and inferior surface of the heart.)
2. The left coronary system and its branches

The major branches of the left coronary system include the left main, which divides into the left anterior descending vessel and feeds the left anterior surface of the heart, and the circumflex branch, which feeds the lateral left ventricle and a portion of the posterior surface of the heart.

Coronary arteries can become obstructed by the development of a clot or the build up of fatty deposits (atherosclerosis). Both conditions cause a heart attack (myocardial infarction [MI]) and require immediate

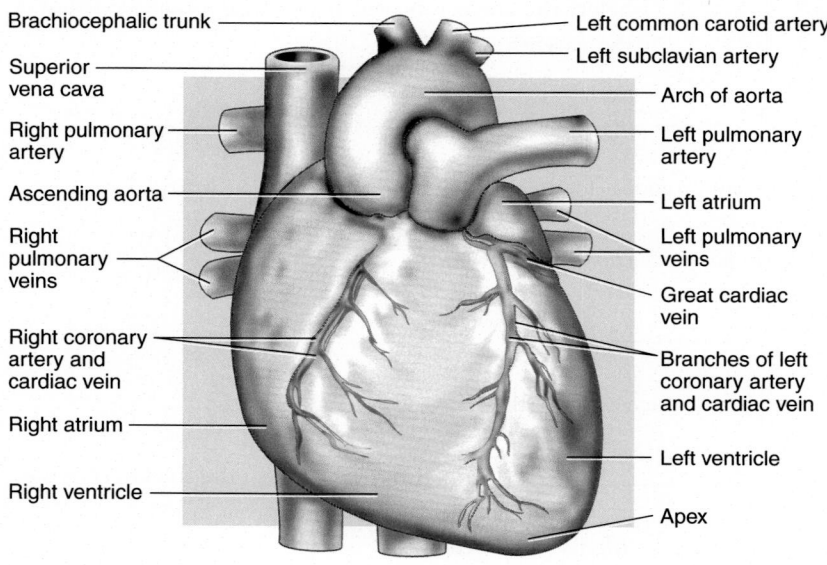

Brachiocephalic trunk
Superior vena cava
Right pulmonary artery
Ascending aorta
Right pulmonary veins
Right coronary artery and cardiac vein
Right atrium
Right ventricle

Left common carotid artery
Left subclavian artery
Arch of aorta
Left pulmonary artery
Left atrium
Left pulmonary veins
Great cardiac vein
Branches of left coronary artery and cardiac vein
Left ventricle
Apex

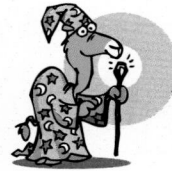

What You NEED TO KNOW

For further information, refer to the *Real World Nursing Survival Guide: Critical Care & Emergency Nursing*.

The right atrium receives venous blood from the systemic circulation, whereas the left atrium receives oxygenated blood from the lungs. Although both atria are filling with blood, the SA node in the electrical conduction system fires and starts the process of depolarization. As the atria fill with blood, the pressure within the atria increases, forcing the AV valves to open. The majority of ventricular filling (diastole) occurs passively when the AV valves open. After atrial depolarization, the atria contract, forcing the remaining atrial blood into the ventricles. This action is referred to as *atrial kick* and contributes as much as 30% of the cardiac output (CO).

Atrial kick = 20%-30% of CO

After atrial contraction, the atria begin to relax and atrial pressure decreases. The electrical impulses from the atria now travel through the remainder of the conduction system and cause ventricular depolarization. This action results in the beginning of ventricular contraction. Ventricular pressure now exceeds atrial pressure, and the AV valves close and the semilunar valves open. Desaturated blood is ejected from the right ventricle into the lungs, where it drops off carbon dioxide and picks up oxygen. Oxygenated blood from the left ventricle is ejected to the systemic circulation via the aorta. The ejection of blood from the ventricles is referred to as systole.

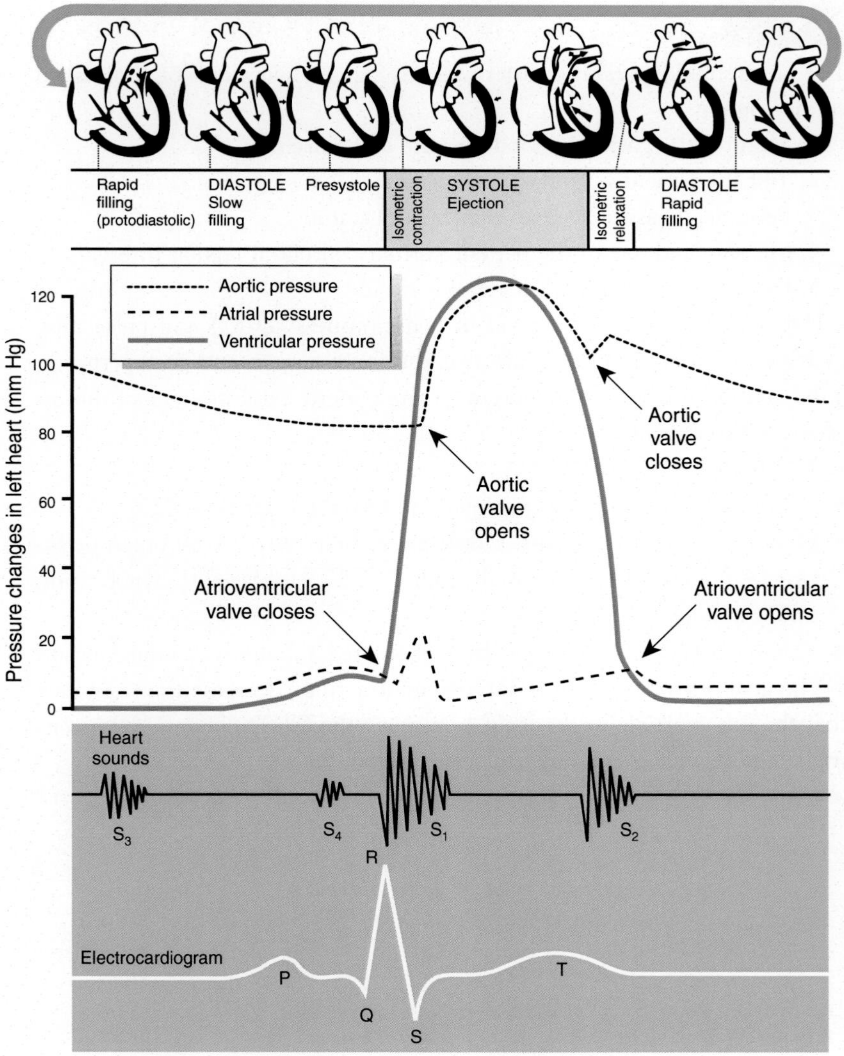

| Rapid filling (protodiastolic) | DIASTOLE Slow filling | Presystole | Isometric contraction | SYSTOLE Ejection | Isometric relaxation | DIASTOLE Rapid filling |

- - - - - - Aortic pressure
- - - Atrial pressure
— Ventricular pressure

Pressure changes in left heart (mm Hg)

120
100
80
60
40
20
0

Aortic valve opens

Aortic valve closes

Atrioventricular valve closes

Atrioventricular valve opens

Heart sounds

S_3 S_4 S_1 S_2

Electrocardiogram

R
P   Q   S   T

Stroke volume is the volume of blood that is ejected during systole. Left ventricular end–**systolic** volume is the amount of blood that remains in the left ventricle at the end of systole. Left ventricular end–**diastolic** volume is the amount of blood that is in the ventricle just before ejection occurs. The left ventricle never ejects the entire volume it receives during diastole. The portion of the volume it does eject is referred to as *ejection fraction*, which is approximately 70% of the total volume at the end of diastole.

TAKE HOME POINTS

Factors that increase contractility are called *positive inotropic agents.* Factors that decrease contractility are referred to as *negative inotropic agents.*

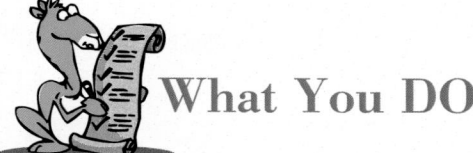

What You DO

The nurse should assess the patient for any signs or symptoms of diminished cardiac output:

1. Monitor the patient's blood pressure and pulse rate.
2. Test the patient's capillary refill time.
3. Periodically assess the patient's mental status.
4. Measure and record the patient's urinary output at regular intervals.
5. Determine the patient's level of perfusion.

Hypotension, changes in level of consciousness (LOC) and pulse rate, increased capillary refill time, decreased urinary output, and poor perfusion indicate diminished cardiac output. If the patient exhibits signs of diminished cardiac output:

- Notify the physician.
- Administer oxygen to keep oxygen saturation greater than 92%.
- Give fluid and vasopressors, if ordered, to help restore vital organ perfusion. A fluid challenge is initially indicated for patients with hypotension and is usually well tolerated.
- Administer positive inotropic drugs, if ordered, to improve cardiac output.

The goal of treatment is to improve contractility, decrease the resistance that the left ventricle works against, improve the filling volume of the ventricle, and regulate heart rate and rhythm.

A fluid challenge can precipitate heart failure and pulmonary edema in the patient who is already volume overloaded.

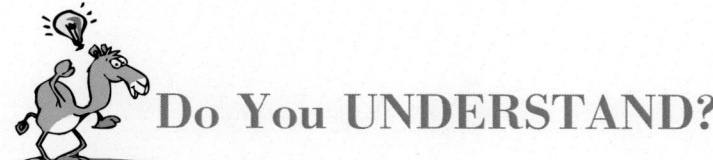

Do You UNDERSTAND?

DIRECTIONS: Fill in the blanks to complete each of the following statements.

1. During systole, the _____ valves are open and

   the _____ valves are closed.

2. During diastole, the _____ valves are open and

   the _____ valves are closed.

3. Atrial contraction is referred to as _____

   _____ and contributes as much as

   _____ % of the cardiac output.

4. The left ventricle never ejects the entire volume it receives during sys-

   tole. The portion of blood that the left ventricle ejects during systole is

   referred to as the _____ _____.

5. The volume of blood that is in the ventricle just before ejection occurs

   is called _____ _____

   _____-_____ _____.

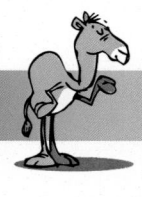

What IS the Anatomy and Physiology of the Pulmonary System (Lungs)?

The pulmonary system facilitates gas exchange of oxygen (O_2) and carbon dioxide (CO_2) between the atmosphere and alveoli. The pulmonary system is made up of the upper airway, lower airway, and lungs. The upper airway provides gas exchange to and from the lower airway; it includes the nose, pharynx, and larynx. The lower airway provides gas exchange to the alveoli and includes the trachea, bronchi, bronchioles, and terminal bronchioles.

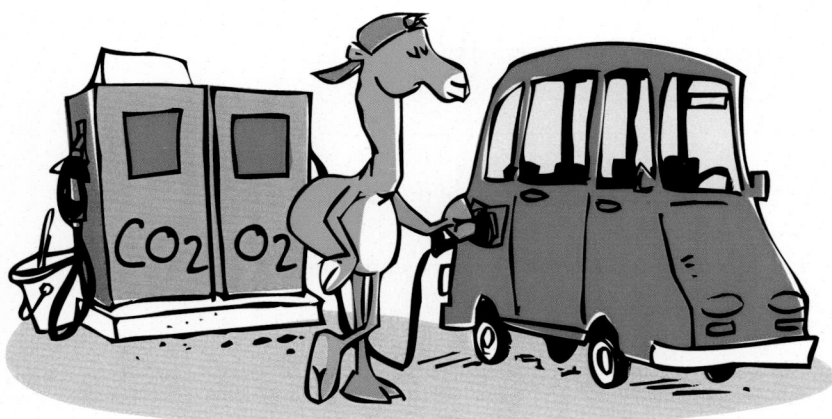

Two lungs exist—the right lung and the left lung. The right lung has three lobes, and the left lung has two. Each lobe contains segments or lobules supplied by one bronchiole. The pleura are the coverings of the lungs, consisting of two layers. The inner layer is referred to as the *visceral pleura,* and the outer layer is called the *parietal pleura.* A space exists between the two pleura that contains a small amount of fluid; it is called the *pleural space.* The pressure in the pleural space is always less than atmospheric pressure (negative pressure), enabling inspiration to occur and lung expansion to be maintained.

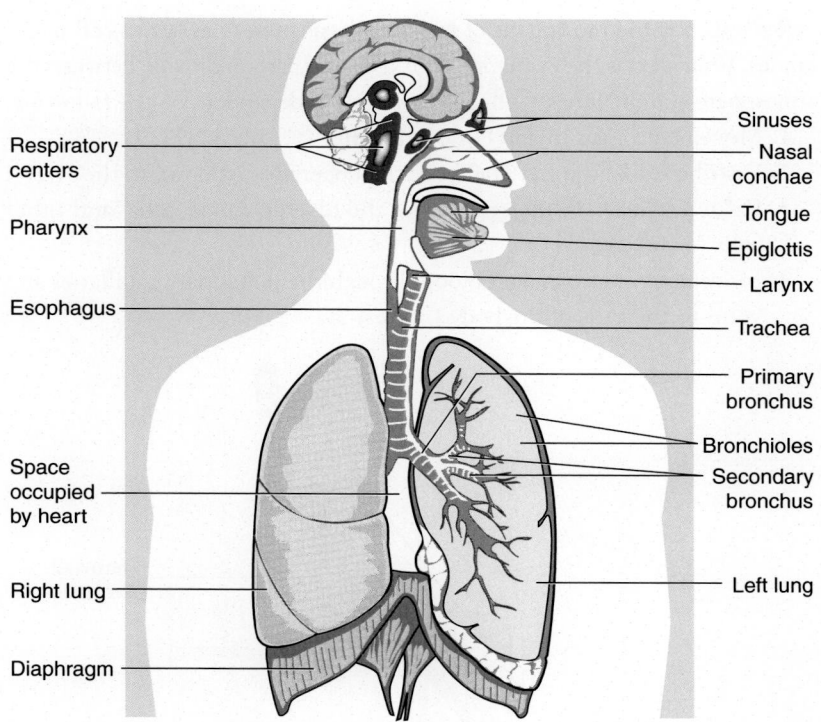

Respiratory centers
Sinuses
Nasal conchae
Pharynx
Tongue
Epiglottis
Larynx
Esophagus
Trachea
Primary bronchus
Bronchioles
Secondary bronchus
Space occupied by heart
Right lung
Left lung
Diaphragm

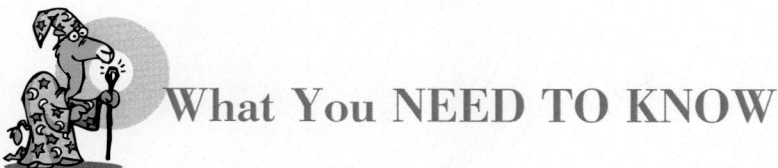

What You NEED TO KNOW

Mechanics of Breathing

Changes in intrapleural pressure, along with pressures in the lungs, result in the process of breathing. In the resting state, intrapleural pressure is less than atmospheric pressure, and the pressure in the alveoli equals atmospheric pressure. With inspiration, the diaphragm lowers and flattens and the intercostal muscles contract, lifting the chest cavity up and out. Therefore both the intrapleural pressure and the alveolar pressure become more negative relative to atmospheric pressure. Because atmospheric pressure is greater, air flows into the lungs. Expiration occurs passively; the diaphragm and intercostal muscles relax causing the lungs to recoil. This action generates a positive alveolar pressure and air flows out of the lungs (expiration). The function of the pulmonary system is to exchange oxygen and carbon dioxide between the air and the cells of the body.

Respiration is the movement of respiratory gas molecules across cell membranes. *Ventilation* is the exchange of oxygen and carbon dioxide between the atmosphere and the lungs. Cellular respiration is dependent on the following:

1. Movement of gas in and out of the lungs (ventilation)
2. Distribution of the gases between the upper airways down to the alveoli
3. Passive transfer of the gases from the alveoli, blood cells, and other cells (diffusion)
4. Movement of oxygenated blood through the pulmonary capillaries and veins to the cells of the body (perfusion)

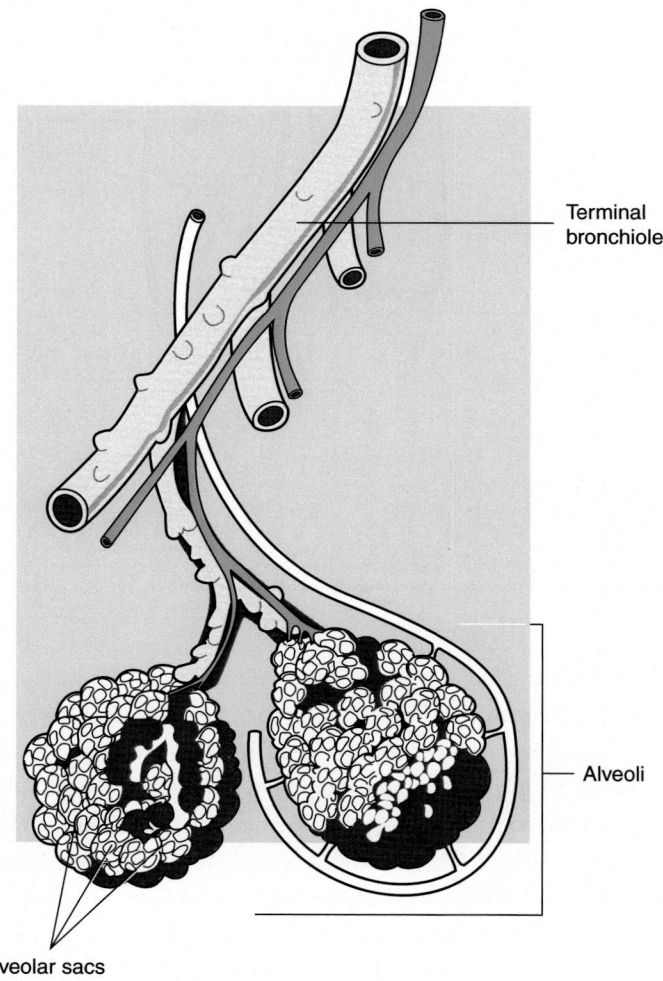

Terminal bronchiole

Alveoli

Alveolar sacs

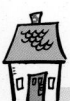

Pulmonary Circulation

Mixed venous blood flows into the main pulmonary artery from the right ventricle. The pulmonary artery divides into two major branches—one to the right lung and one to the left lung. These arteries continue dividing until they become arterioles and join in the capillary network surrounding each alveolus. This network of capillaries and arterioles has thin walls that are very elastic, allowing low systolic and diastolic pulmonary pressures.

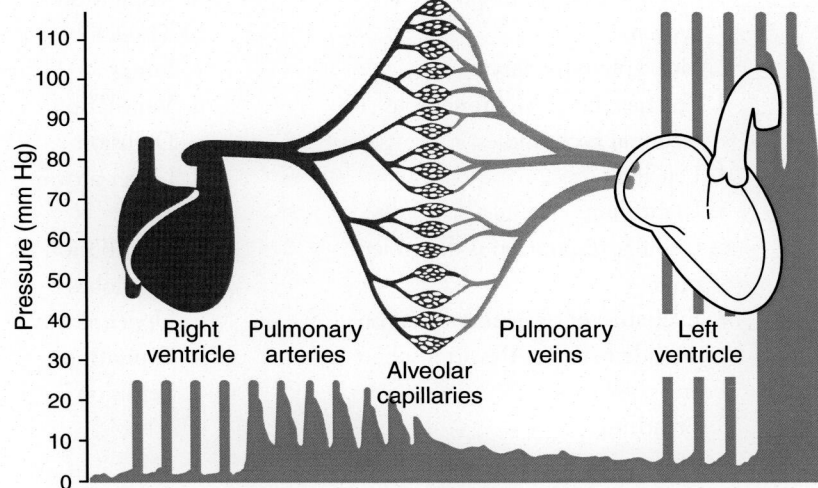

PULMONARY CHANGES WITH THE AGING PATIENT

- Decreased elasticity of chest wall
- Decreased alveolar surface area
- Increased rigidity of chest wall
- Increased weakness of respiratory muscles
- Increased risk for pneumonia, poor gas exchange, respiratory distress, and respiratory failure

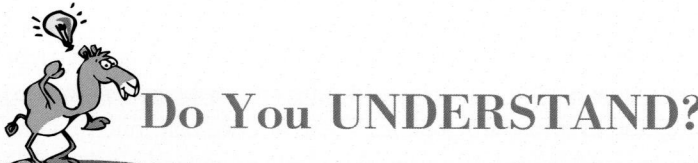

Do You UNDERSTAND?

DIRECTIONS: **Match each phrase in Column A with the appropriate phrase or phrases in Column B.**

Column A

_____ 1. Components of the pulmonary system

_____ 2. Nose, pharynx, larynx

_____ 3. Trachea, bronchi, bronchioles, terminal bronchioles

_____ 4. Left lung

_____ 5. Right lung

_____ 6. Cellular respiration is dependent on it

_____ 7. Exchange of oxygen and carbon dioxide between the atmosphere and the lungs

_____ 8. Breathing

_____ 9. Movement of gas in and out of the lungs

_____ 10. Occurs passively, generating positive alveolar pressure

Column B

a. Inspiration
b. Three lobes
c. Lungs
d. Ventilation
e. Diffusion
f. Lower airway
g. Heart
h. Distribution
i. Two lobes
j. Upper airway
k. Expiration
l. Perfusion

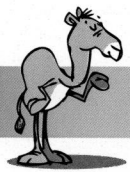

What IS Pulmonary Vascular Resistance?

The right ventricle must overcome pressure to promote the forward flow of blood through the pulmonary circulation. This pressure is called *pulmonary vascular resistance* (PVR). PVR is affected by the elasticity of the pulmonary arteries, capillaries, and veins. Because of high distensibility of the pulmonary vasculature, the PVR is normally low. However, when pulmonary arterioles become constricted, PVR increases. Conversely, if the arterioles dilate, then PVR decreases.

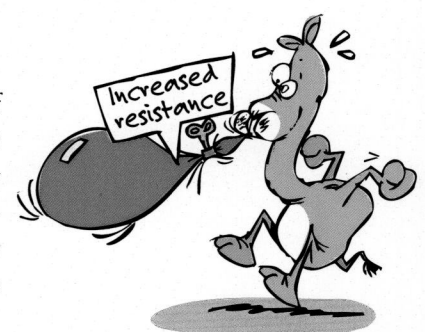

Answers: 1. c, f; 2. j; 3. f; 4. i; 5. b; 6. d, e, h, l; 7. d; 8. a, k; 9. d; 10. k.

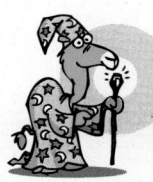

What You NEED TO KNOW

PVR may increase or decrease as a result of pulmonary disease or vasoactive agents or because of other influences such as the autonomic nervous system. Sympathetic stimulation causes a slight increase in PVR, and parasympathetic stimulation causes minimal pulmonary vessel dilation and slight decreases in resistance. Vasoconstrictive agents can increase PVR and elevate pulmonary artery systolic and diastolic pressures. Dilator drugs lower resistance and pulmonary artery pressures.

Decreased oxygen in the blood (hypoxemia) causes pulmonary capillary vasoconstriction and increases resistance. Acidosis also causes vasoconstriction, along with increased carbon dioxide levels in the blood (hypercapnea), which results in increased PVR.

The collapse of alveoli or parts of lung tissue is called *atelectasis*. Usually this collapse occurs as a result of mucous plugs or partially obstructed airways. Atelectasis causes compression of pulmonary capillaries, arteries, and veins, which increases resistance.

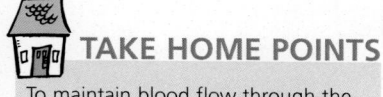

TAKE HOME POINTS

To maintain blood flow through the lungs and appropriate filling of the left heart, pulmonary artery systolic and diastolic pressures increase in proportion to the increase in PVR.

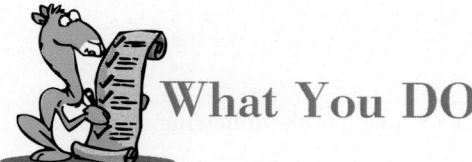

What You DO

- Assess the patient for signs and symptoms of diminished oxygenation.

SIGNS AND SYMPTOMS OF DIMINISHED OXYGENATION
• Shortness of breath (dyspnea)
• Increase in respiratory rate (tachypnea)
• Increase in heart rate (tachycardia)
• Increase in the work of breathing (use of accessory muscles)
• Changes in LOC
• Changes in color (cyanosis)
• Increased capillary refill time (greater than 3 seconds)

- Notify the physician immediately if the patient exhibits signs of respiratory distress or diminished oxygenation.
- Monitor the patient's oxygen saturation, and administer oxygen to keep the patient's oxygen saturation above 92%.

- Assess the patient for signs of right ventricular dysfunction.

SIGNS AND SYMPTOMS OF RIGHT VENTRICULAR DYSFUNCTION

- Distended neck veins
- Dependent pitting edema
- Increased fatigue
- Hepatomegaly
- Ascites

- Weight gain
- Increased frequency of urination after lying in bed (**nocturia**)
- Elevated central venous pressures (right atrial and right ventricular pressures)

- Position the patient to facilitate breathing (semi-Fowler position).
- Closely monitor the patient's intake and output.
- Monitor the patient's daily weights.
- Observe fluid and sodium restrictions.
- Monitor the patient's electrolytes and arterial blood gases (ABGs).
- Observe the patient for any changes of worsening failure (e.g., increased shortness of breath, pulmonary congestion, increasing tachycardia).
- Administer medications including diuretics, vasodilators, and positive inotropes as ordered.

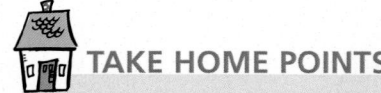

TAKE HOME POINTS

Acute and chronic changes in the pulmonary circuit can profoundly affect cardiac function and hemodynamic status.

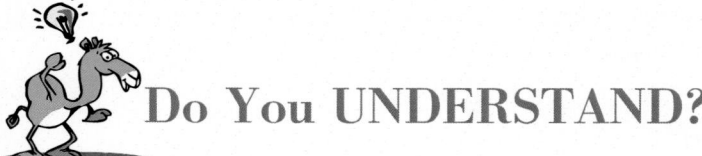

Do You UNDERSTAND?

DIRECTIONS: Fill in the blanks to complete the following statements.

1. The pressure that the right ventricle must overcome to promote forward flow of blood through pulmonary circulation is referred to as

_____

_____ _____.

2. Three factors may alter PVR. They are:

_____

_____

_____

2 Hemodynamic Theory

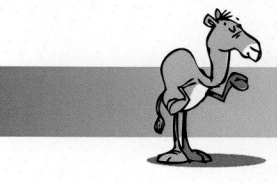

What IS the Relationship of the Circulatory System, the Heart, and Hemodynamics?

Hemodynamics is the study of forces involved in blood flow through the cardiovascular and circulatory systems. The components of hemodynamics include blood pressure (BP), central venous pressure (CVP), and right and left heart pressures.

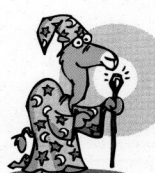

What You NEED TO KNOW

The physiologic principles of hemodynamics include factors that affect myocardial function, the regulation of BP, the determination of cardiac performance, and cardiac output (CO). Understanding the basic concepts of pressure, flow, and resistance provide an insight into understanding hemodynamic theory. Assessing ventricular function through the use of hemodynamic variables enables the nurse to identify cardiovascular problems, to determine appropriate interventions, and to assess outcomes that optimize the delivery of oxygen (O_2) to tissues.

Circulatory System

The flow of blood through the circulatory system is regulated by several mechanisms. When the metabolic demands of the body increase, the blood vessels constrict, forcing blood back to the heart. When the metabolic demand decreases, the veins dilate. This dilation causes pooling of blood in the peripheral veins and reduces venous return to the heart. Other mechanisms that control flow result from the ability of the heart to increase or decrease its rate and strength of contraction.

Pulmonary Artery

The pulmonary artery is the blood vessel that carries desaturated blood from the right ventricle to the lungs. When monitoring hemodynamic pressures, the catheter that measures pulmonary artery pressures is placed in the pulmonary artery. This catheter can measure pressures in the pulmonary artery, pulmonary capillary bed, left atrium, and, during diastole, the left ventricle.

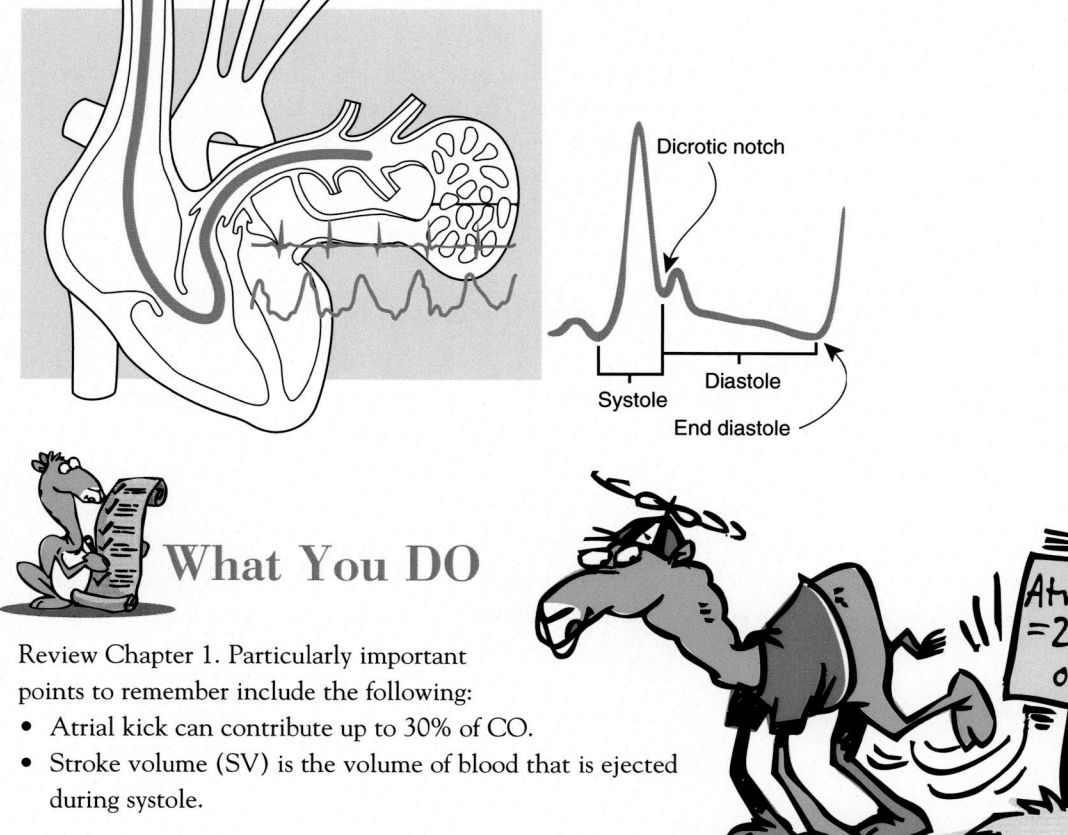

Dicrotic notch

Systole

Diastole

End diastole

What You DO

Review Chapter 1. Particularly important points to remember include the following:

- Atrial kick can contribute up to 30% of CO.
- Stroke volume (SV) is the volume of blood that is ejected during systole.

- Left ventricular end–systolic volume is the amount of blood that remains in the left ventricle at the end of systole.
- Left ventricular end–diastolic volume is the amount of blood that is in the ventricle just before ejection (systole) occurs.
- The left ventricle never ejects the entire volume it receives during diastole.
- The portion of the volume it does eject is referred to as ejection fraction, which is approximately 70% of the total volume at the end of diastole.

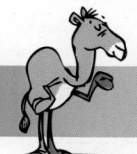

Do You UNDERSTAND?

DIRECTIONS: Identify the following statements as *true* (T) or *false* (F).

_____ 1. During systole the semilunar valves are open and the atrioventricular (AV) valves are closed.

_____ 2. Atrial kick is responsible for as much as a 40% contribution to CO.

_____ 3. The ventricular end–diastolic volume is the portion of blood the right ventricle ejects during diastole.

_____ 4. The heart pumps a constant volume of blood.

_____ 5. The cardiac conduction system provides electrical activation to cause the heart to contract.

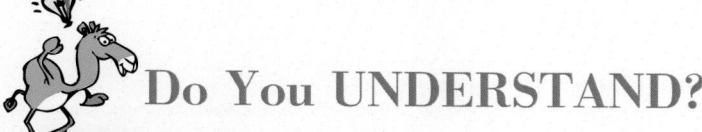

What IS Blood Pressure?

BP is defined as the tension exerted by blood on the arterial walls.

  BP = resistance × flow

Peripheral vascular resistance (PVR) and CO directly affect BP. If a patient's BP decreases, either the flow (CO) or systemic vascular resistance (SVR) has changed. Narrowed vessels increase both resistance and BP. Conversely, dilated vessels decrease resistance and BP.

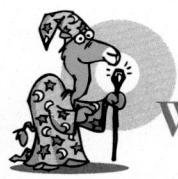

What You NEED TO KNOW

 For further information, visit National Heart, Lung and Blood Institute, National Institute of Health at www.nhlbi.nih.gov/guidelines/ hypertension.

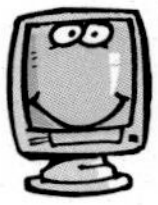

Monitoring of BP is based on the following equation:

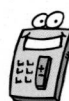 $$BP = CO \times SVR$$

Blood Pressure Values

LEVEL	SBP	DBP
Normal	Less than 120 mm Hg	Less than 80 mm Hg
Prehypertension	120-139 mm Hg	80-89 mm Hg
Hypertension, stage 1	140-159 mm Hg	90-99 mm Hg
Hypertension, stage 2	Greater than 160 mm Hg	Greater than 100 mm Hg

SBP, Systolic blood pressure; *DBP,* diastolic blood pressure.

Factors Influencing Arterial Blood Pressure

```
Mean arterial blood pressure
 ├─ Peripheral resistance
 │    ├─ Blood viscosity (influenced by hematocrit)
 │    └─ Arteriolar lumen size (influenced by sympathetic nervous system)
 ├─ Autonomic control
 └─ Cardiac output
      ├─ Heart rate
      │    └─ Sympathetic and parasympathetic nervous system
      └─ Stroke volume
           └─ Left ventricular end–diastolic volume (preload)
                └─ Intraventricular pressure
                     ├─ Autonomic control
                     ├─ Atrial pressure
                     ├─ Venous pressure
                     │    ├─ Blood volume
                     │    └─ Renin-angiotensin system
                     └─ Venous return
```

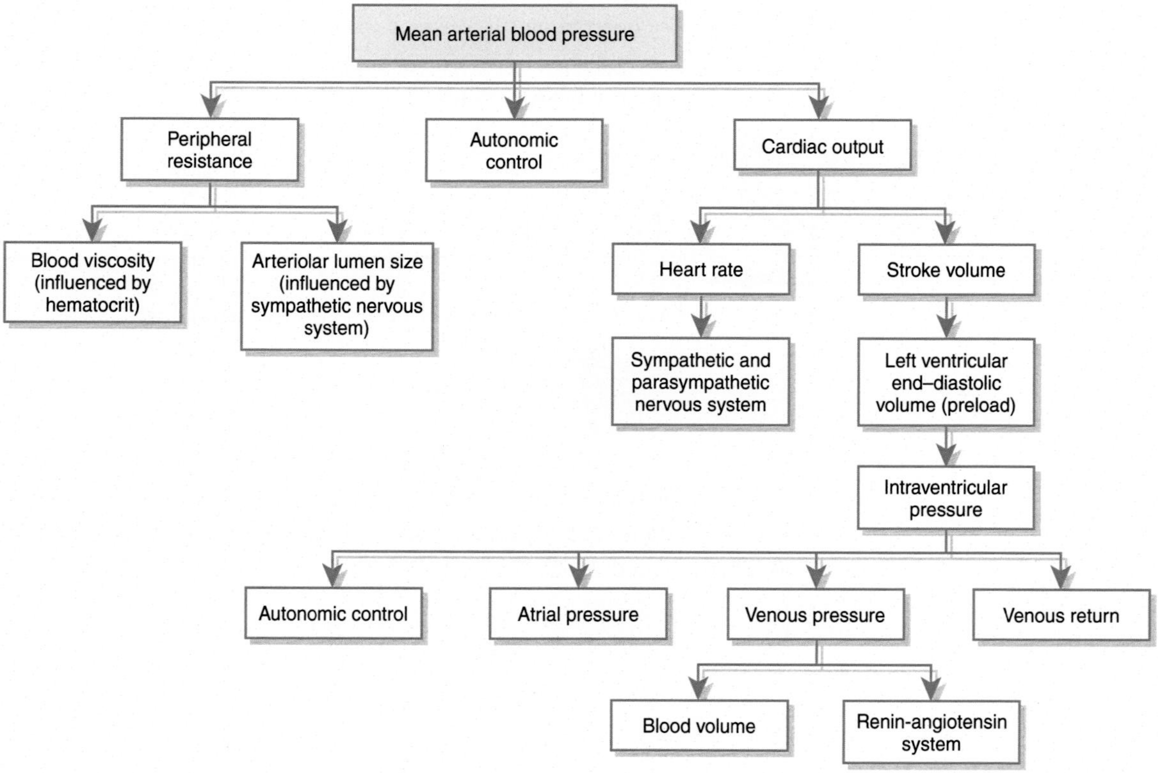

Systemic Vascular Resistance

SVR is a reflection of peripheral vascular resistance and is the opposition to blood flow from the blood vessels. SVR is affected by the tone of the blood vessels, blood viscosity, and resistance from the inner lining of the blood vessels.

SVR is the resistance against which the left ventricle pumps and usually has an inverse relationship with CO. If the SVR decreases, then the CO increases. SVR increases to maintain BP when CO decreases.

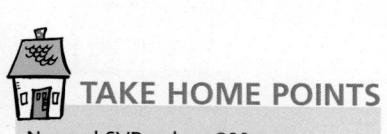

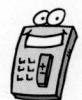

$$SVR = \frac{\text{mean arterial pressure (MAP)} - CVP \times 80}{CO}$$

The diameter of the blood vessel is one of the major factors that influence SVR. SVR decreases when blood vessels relax and increases when blood vessels narrow. Vasoactive drugs are often used in the critical care setting to change the size of the arterioles to decrease or increase BP.

Elevations of SVR increase the workload of the heart and myocardial oxygen consumption. The two primary reasons for elevations in systemic vascular resistance are the following:

1. Hypertension or excessive catecholamine release causes vascular disturbances such as vasoconstriction.
2. Compensatory responses maintain BP in decreased CO.

Several potential causes of decreased SVR exist. These causes include sepsis and neurologic-mediated vasomotor tone loss. When SVR decreases, CO increases in an attempt to maintain BP.

Cardiac Output

CO is the amount of blood ejected from the heart in 1 minute. CO has two components: SV and heart rate (HR). A major goal in assessing CO is ensuring adequate oxygenation.

TAKE HOME POINTS

Normal SVR value: 800 to 1400 dynes/sec/cm^{-5}

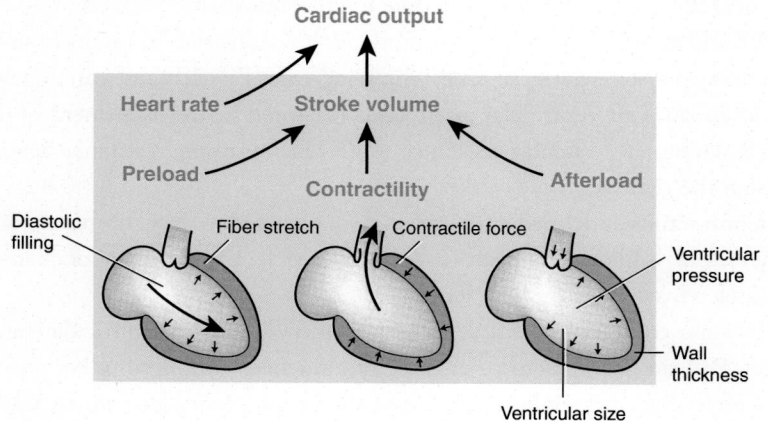

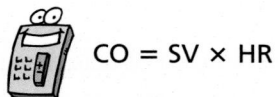

$$CO = SV \times HR$$

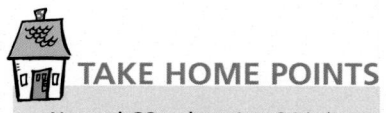

Stroke Volume

SV is the amount of blood ejected from the heart with each beat. Preload, afterload, and contractility are three factors that influence SV.

Preload is the filling volume of the ventricle at the end of diastole (left ventricular end–diastolic volume); however, instead of measuring a volume, pressure is measured. This pressure is called *left ventricular end–diastolic pressure*. It reflects the amount of cardiac muscle stretch at the end diastole, just before contraction. Preload is dependent on the volume of blood returning to the heart. Venous tone and the actual amount of blood in the venous system influence this volume. Preload is measured by obtaining a pressure measurement with a pulmonary artery catheter. This measurement is referred to as a *pulmonary artery occlusion pressure/pulmonary artery wedge pressure/ pulmonary capillary wedge pressure* (PAOP/PAWP/PCWP). Preload is directly related to the force of myocardial stretch and contraction.

Afterload is the amount of resistance against which the ventricle pumps.

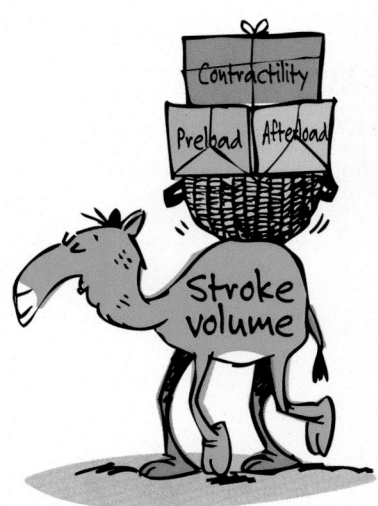

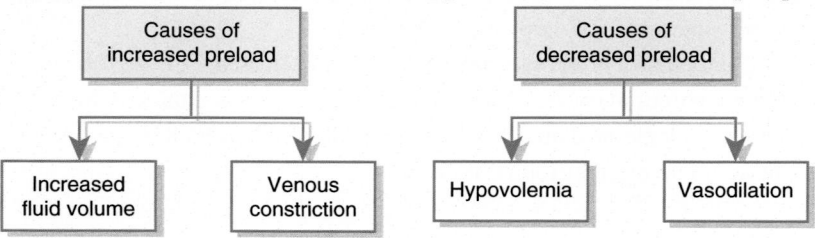

It is primarily influenced by the blood vessels, but blood viscosity, flow patterns, and valves can have an effect. The greater the resistance, the more the myocardium has to work to overcome the resistance.

BP and arterial tone determine afterload. Vasoconstriction results from an increase in systemic arterial tone, which increases BP and causes an increase in afterload. Left ventricular afterload is measured by the assessment of the SVR. Pulmonary vascular resistance (PVR) measures the resistance against which the right ventricle works.

Contractility is defined as the strength of myocardial fiber shortening during systole. It allows the heart to work independently, regardless of changes in preload, afterload, or fiber length.

Because contractility is a determinant of SV, it affects ventricular function. Preload is one factor that directly influences contractility because of the physiologic principle referred to as the *Frank-Starling law*, which states, "The greater the stretch, the greater the force of the next contraction."

Increases in preload (end-diastolic volume) can maximally increase SV. However, relationships are not directly linear in cases of compromised cardiac or pulmonary function, volume, and pressure. As resistance to left ventricular ejection (afterload) increases, left ventricular work increases and SV may decrease. The ventricular stroke work index (VSWI) is a useful measurement of myocardial contractility.

$$\text{Left VSWI} = \text{MAP} - \text{PCWP} \times \text{stroke volume index (SVI)} \times 0.0136$$

$$\text{SVI} = \text{SV} \div \text{body surface area (BSA)}$$

Heart Rate

The number of heartbeats per minute is important in maintaining CO and is included in the CO formula. When contractility is depressed or if CO is decreased, then the HR increases to maintain sufficient blood flow for metabolic demand. An increased HR (tachycardia) decreases diastolic filling time, which decreases fiber stretch and can decrease the volume of blood ejected with each beat. A slower HR (bradycardia) increases diastolic filling time, which can allow overstretching or filling of the ventricles.

However, remember that the formula for CO is:

Manipulation of Cardiac Output (CO = SV × HR)

FACTORS AFFECTING STROKE VOLUME (preload, afterload, contractility)	
PROBLEM	**INTERVENTIONS**
Increased preload	• Diuretics
	• Venodilators
Decreased preload	• Fluids
	• Vasoconstrictors
Increased SVR	• Arterial vasodilators
Decrease SVR	• Vasoconstrictors
Increased contractility	• Negative inotropes
Decreased contractility	• Positives inotropes
Increased heart rate	• Beta blockers
	• Calcium channel blockers
Decreased heart rate	• Sympathometic drugs
	• Cardiac pacing

CO, Cardiac output; *SV,* stroke volume; *HR,* heart rate; *SVR,* systemic vascular resistance.

$$\text{CO} = \text{SV} \times \text{HR}$$

Therefore changes in HR can be a compensatory mechanism to increase CO.

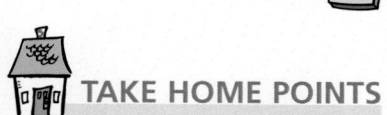

TAKE HOME POINTS

Left VSWI normal value: 35 to 85gm/m²/beat

SVI normal value: 30 to 65 ml/beat/m²

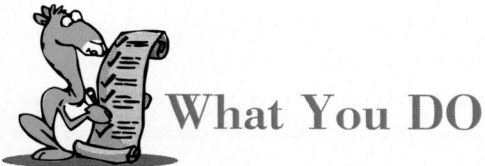

What You DO

To regulate hemodynamic parameters, the nurse should take steps to maintain BP and adequate SV, HR, and rhythm.

Maintaining Blood Pressure

The goal of treatment for hypertension is to prevent death and complications by lowering and maintaining the patient's BP. Treatment includes risk factor and lifestyle modification, reduction of body weight, decreased dietary sodium, increased physical activity, moderation of alcohol consumption, stress management, and smoking cessation.

In malignant **hyper**tension, BP is sufficiently elevated to cause acute vascular injury in vital organs. The goal of treatment is to lower the BP slowly, over 6 to 24 hours. Treatment may be initiated with intravenous antihypertensive agents.

Hypotension with signs or symptoms such as dizziness, change in level of consciousness (LOC), and decreased urinary output is first treated with a fluid bolus of 250 to 500 ml of normal saline. Vasopressors are given if BP levels cannot be maintained with fluid bolus.

Maintaining Adequate Stroke Volume

To maintain adequate SV (preload, afterload, and contractility), the nurse should remember these points:
- Fluids increase preload; diuretics decrease preload.
- Vasopressors increase SVR; vasodilators decrease SVR.
- Positive inotropes **increase** contractility; negative inotropes **decrease** contractility.

Maintaining Adequate Heart Rate and Rhythm

To maintain adequate HR and rhythm, the nurse should remember these points:
- Drugs that can increase HR include atropine and sympathomimetics.
- Drugs that can decrease HR include beta blockers and calcium channel blockers.
- Antiarrhythmic drugs can help maintain a regular heart rhythm.
- Cardiac pacing can help maintain rate and rhythm.

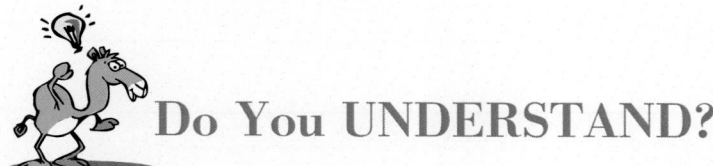

Do You UNDERSTAND?

DIRECTIONS: **Fill in the blanks to complete each of the following statements.**

1. The formula for BP is: _____ × _____.

2. Three factors that influence SV are (1) _____,

   (2) _____, and (3) _____.

3. PAWP, also called _____, is a reflection of

   _____ _____

   _____ – _____ _____.

4. Preload is directly related to the force of myocardial _____

   and _____.

5. CO = _____ × _____.

6. Preload, afterload, and contractility are determinants of

   _____ _____.

7. Preload is defined as _____

   _____

   _____.

8. Afterload is defined as the _____

   _____

   _____.

9. PCWP measures _____.

10. SVR measures _____.

11. The strength of myocardial fiber shortening during systole is referred to

    as _____.

DIRECTIONS: **Match the descriptions in Column A with the terms in Column B.**

Column A	Column B
_____ 12. Increased SVR	a. Sepsis, vasomotor tone loss
_____ 13. Decreased SVR	
_____ 14. The resistance the right ventricle works against.	b. vasoconstriction, compensatory responses
_____ 15. The resistance the left ventricle works against.	c. SVR
	d. PVR

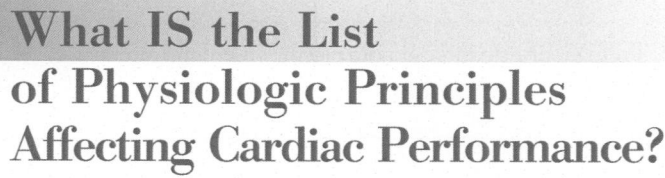

What IS the List of Physiologic Principles Affecting Cardiac Performance?

Factors that influence cardiac performance include the Frank-Starling law of the heart, the ability to influence contractility of the muscle fibers of the heart (inotropism), any changes in HR or regularity of rhythm, and miscellaneous influences such as responses of the sympathetic and parasympathetic nervous systems.

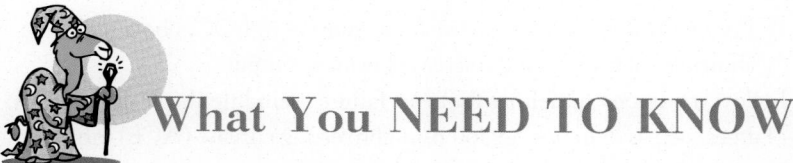

What You NEED TO KNOW

As previously discussed, the Frank-Starling law of the heart states, "The greater the stretch, the greater the force of the next contraction." Augmenting ventricular filling during diastole before the onset of contraction will increase the force of contraction during systole.

Inotropism is the ability to influence contractility of muscle fibers. A positive inotrope enhances contractility. A negative inotrope depresses contractility.

Any change in HR or rhythm (force-frequency ratio) can change the diastolic filling time of the ventricles, thereby altering fiber stretch and the force of the next contraction. This action will influence SV and CO. Additionally, the majority of coronary artery filling occurs during diastole. When HRs increase, myocardial oxygen demand increases. However, diastolic filling time is shortened, thereby decreasing coronary artery filling. This action results in an imbalance between myocardial oxygen supply and demand. Factors such as hypoxia, hyperkalemia, hypercarbia, hyponatremia, and myocardial scar tissue can decrease myocardial contractility. Sympathetic stimulation increases myocardial contractility and parasympathetic stimulation (via the vagus nerve) and depresses the sinoatrial (SA) node, atrial myocardium, and AV junctional tissue.

Heart failure, pulmonary edema, and cardiogenic shock can result if myocardial contractility is decreased as a result of significant damage of the myocardium.

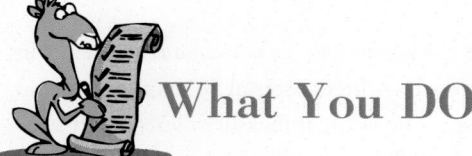

What You DO

Changes in the parameters that affect cardiac performance alter the hemodynamic status of the patient. The nurse should:

- Monitor the patient for the following signs and symptoms of heart failure and poor perfusion:
    1. Left ventricular failure, including tachycardia, dyspnea, pulmonary crackles, and restlessness as a result of hypoxemia
    2. Right ventricular failure, including jugular venous distention, peripheral edema, and hepatomegaly

3. Poor perfusion, which may include changes in LOC, chest pain, shortness of breath, and decreased urinary output

- Follow treatment guidelines for heart failure including the administration of drugs such as diuretics, angiotensin-converting enzyme (ACE) inhibitors, inotropic agents, and beta-adrenergic blockers.

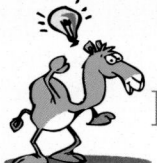

Do You UNDERSTAND?

DIRECTIONS: **Match the descriptions in Column A with the terms in Column B.**

Column A	Column B
_____ 1. Decreases myocardial contractility	a. Sympathetic stimulation
	b. Influencing contraction
_____ 2. Increases myocardial contractility	c. Frank-Starling law
	d. Hypoxia, hypercarbia, hyperkalemia, hyponatremia
_____ 3. Inotropism	
_____ 4. "The greater the stretch, the greater the next force of contraction."	

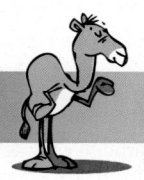

What IS Hemodynamic Monitoring?

Hemodynamics or pressures of the cardiovascular and circulatory system can be measured by invasive methods, such as direct arterial BP monitoring and central venous pressure monitoring, or by indirect measurements of left ventricular pressures via a flow-directed, balloon-tipped catheter.

The goals of hemodynamic monitoring include ensuring adequate perfusion, detecting inadequate perfusion, titrating therapy to a specific endpoint, qualifying the severity of illness, and differentiating system dysfunction (i.e., differentiating between cardiogenic and noncardiogenic pulmonary edema).

Answers: 1. d; 2. a; 3. b; 4. c.

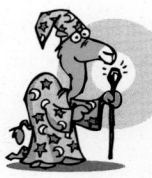

What You NEED TO KNOW

Direct Arterial Blood Pressure Monitoring

Direct intraarterial monitoring allows for accurate, continuous monitoring of arterial BPs. It also provides a system for continuous sampling of blood for arterial blood gases (ABGs) without repeated arterial punctures. Clinical considerations include the potential complications of thrombosis, embolism, blood loss, and infection. Invasive intraarterial monitoring is considered to be more accurate and reliable than noninvasive types of BP monitoring. (Refer to Chapter 4 for more information on arterial pressure monitoring.)

Right Atrial Pressure Monitoring

Measurement of pressures from the right atrium can be referred to right atrial pressure (RAP) or CVP. This measurement of pressure is taken directly from the superior or inferior vena cava (CVP) or from the right atrium (RAP). The pressures between these two areas are essentially equal. Because the tricuspid valve (AV valve between the right atrium and right ventricle) is open during diastole, a RAP measurement can reliably reflect right ventricular end–diastolic pressure.

Any condition that changes venous tone, blood volume, or contractility of the right ventricle can cause an abnormality in RAP values. Low RAP measurements can reflect hypovolemia or extreme vasodilation. High RAP measurements can be reflective of hypervolemia or severe vasoconstriction. Additionally, conditions that reduce the ability of the right ventricle to eject, such as pulmonary hypertension and right ventricular failure, can elevate RAP.

Left Atrial Pressure Monitoring

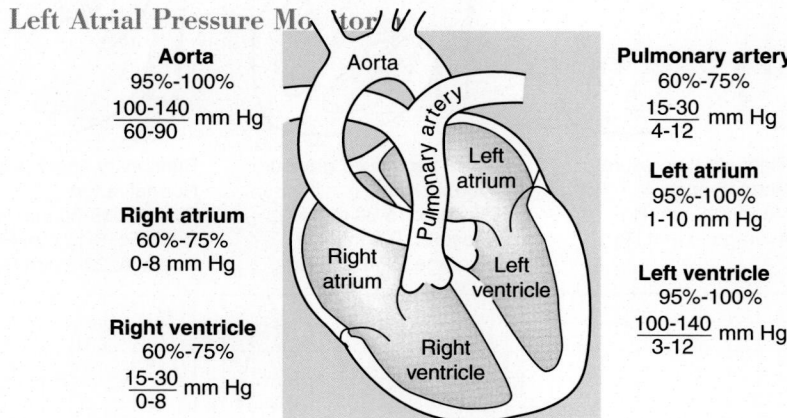

Aorta
95%-100%
$\frac{100\text{-}140}{60\text{-}90}$ mm Hg

Right atrium
60%-75%
0-8 mm Hg

Right ventricle
60%-75%
$\frac{15\text{-}30}{0\text{-}8}$ mm Hg

Pulmonary artery
60%-75%
$\frac{15\text{-}30}{4\text{-}12}$ mm Hg

Left atrium
95%-100%
1-10 mm Hg

Left ventricle
95%-100%
$\frac{100\text{-}140}{3\text{-}12}$ mm Hg

Aorta, Pulmonary artery, Left atrium, Right atrium, Left ventricle, Right ventricle

Left atrial pressure (LAP) monitoring directly measures pressures in the left atrium of the heart. Direct LAP monitoring is not routinely used except in cardiac surgical procedures, in cardiac catheterization laboratories, and in cardiac surgical units. Most often, a catheter is inserted during cardiac surgery with the distal end tunneled through an incision in the chest wall. LAP monitoring provides the ability to observe the pressures in the left atrium. However, air embolism or system debris, which can obstruct a coronary or cerebral artery, can be a major complication.

Pulmonary Artery Pressure Monitoring

Pulmonary artery pressure monitoring measures pressures in the pulmonary artery, reflecting left ventricular end–diastolic pressure. The pulmonary artery catheter is a multilumen, balloon-tipped catheter that is inserted through the venous system into the right heart and pulmonary artery. The catheter may be inserted at the bedside from an antecubital, an external jugular, a subclavian, or other peripheral vein into the pulmonary artery through a percutaneous introducer. Fluoroscopy is not required because the pressure tracing on the monitor can identify its positioning. The catheter is inserted with the balloon deflated. When the catheter enters the right atrium, the balloon is inflated, allowing it to float with the flow of blood into the pulmonary artery. When the balloon is deflated, the catheter directly measures pulmonary artery pressures. With balloon inflation, the catheter floats into a pulmonary arteriole and wedges itself in a smaller lumen. The opening of the catheter beyond the inflated balloon reflects pressures distal to the pulmonary artery.

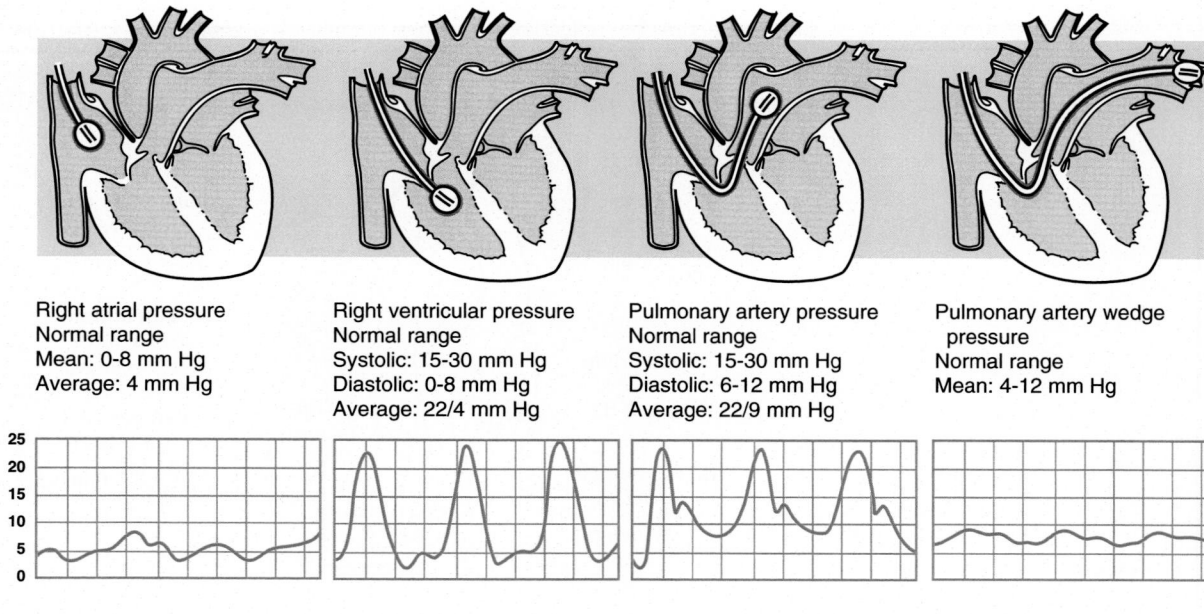

Right atrial pressure
Normal range
Mean: 0-8 mm Hg
Average: 4 mm Hg

Right ventricular pressure
Normal range
Systolic: 15-30 mm Hg
Diastolic: 0-8 mm Hg
Average: 22/4 mm Hg

Pulmonary artery pressure
Normal range
Systolic: 15-30 mm Hg
Diastolic: 6-12 mm Hg
Average: 22/9 mm Hg

Pulmonary artery wedge
 pressure
Normal range
Mean: 4-12 mm Hg

This PCWP, also referred to as the PAOP, indirectly measures left ventricular function because the mean PCWP or PAOP and left atrial pressures closely approximate left ventricular end–diastolic pressure in patients with normal mitral valve function.

It is important to remember that changes in PCWP are not always equal to volume changes because the PCWP is not the only parameter involved in muscle stretch. Patients who have compliant left ventricles can have large volume changes without large changes in pressure. Conversely, patients with noncompliant ventricles may have extreme volume changes with PCWP increases.

The proximal lumen of the catheter allows for the monitoring of CVPs. A cable can attach the thermistor port to a CO computer, allowing monitoring of CO. From this port, baseline blood temperature is obtained, as well as a thermal CO curve and digital readout of CO. (See Chapter 8 for further information on CO.)

Pulmonary artery catheters may also have additional lumens, which allow for intravenous administration of solutions or insertion of pacemaker electrodes for the purpose of transvenous pacing.

Other catheters also have the ability to monitor CO or mixed venous oxygen saturation on a continuous basis. The pulmonary artery catheter is used to monitor high-risk, critically ill patients with the goals of detecting adequate perfusion and diagnosis and evaluation of the effects of therapy. This patient group includes those with a variety of cardiopulmonary problems (e.g., acute myocardial infarction, severe angina, cardiomyopathy, right and left ventricular failure, pulmonary disease). The pulmonary artery catheter is also a valuable tool for monitoring fluid balance in the critically ill, high-risk patient.

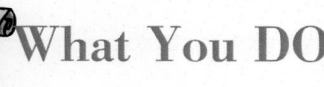

What You DO

To monitor hemodynamics, the following equipment must be gathered first:

- Transducer
- Amplifier
- Display monitor
- Catheter system
- Noncompliant pressure tubing
- Normal saline
- Pressure bag

The hemodynamic monitoring system and setup provides the ability to monitor a pressure waveform and digital readout of the pressure being monitored.

Nursing interventions for hemodynamic monitoring include the following:

🍎 Teach the patient about the procedure.

- Obtain the patient's signature on the appropriate procedure consent forms.

- Set up the equipment, prepare and zero the line, and assist the physician with catheter insertion.
- Monitor the pressures and therapies per institutional policy.
- Monitor the patient for potential complications.

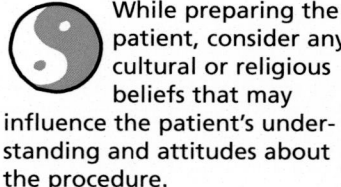

While preparing the patient, consider any cultural or religious beliefs that may influence the patient's understanding and attitudes about the procedure.

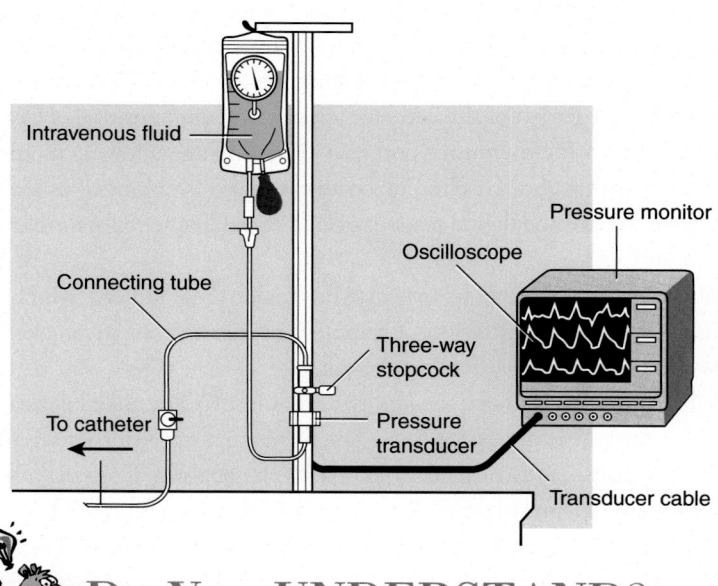

Intravenous fluid

Pressure monitor

Oscilloscope

Connecting tube

Three-way stopcock

To catheter

Pressure transducer

Transducer cable

Do You UNDERSTAND?

DIRECTIONS: List five goals of hemodynamic monitoring.

1. _____

2. _____

3. _____

4. _____

5. _____

Answers: 1. Ensure adequate perfusion; 2. Detect inadequate perfusion; 3. Titrate therapy to a specific endpoint; 4. Differentiate between cardiogenic and noncardiogenic pulmonary edema; 5. Determine the severity of illness.

DIRECTIONS: **Fill in the blanks to complete each of the following statements.**

6. Direct intraarterial monitoring allows for monitoring of

   ________________________ and ________________________

   ________________________ ________________________.

7. CVP measures pressure in the ________________________

   ________________________.

8. Pulmonary artery pressure monitoring measures pulmonary artery

   ________________________, ________________________,

   and ________________________ pressures.

9. With balloon inflation, the catheter floats into a smaller pulmonary arteriole and "wedges." This pressure is referred to by the abbreviation

   ________________________ or ________________________.

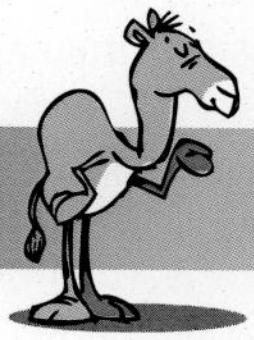

What IS the Relationship of Oxygen Supply and Demand on Hemodynamic Variables?

When assessing hemodynamic variables for the purpose of clinical decision making, the components of oxygen supply and demand must be considered. All living cells require oxygen for cellular work. Without it, a major shift in metabolism occurs, which promotes the production of lactic acid. This acidosis advances a continuous cycle of anaerobic metabolism and further acidosis.

Answers: 6. continuous, accurate blood pressures; 7. right atrium; 8. systolic, diastolic, mean; 9. PCWP, PAOP.

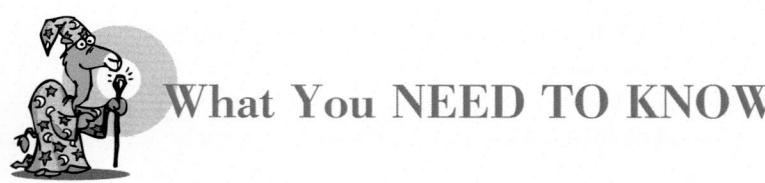

What You NEED TO KNOW

Oxygen Delivery

Oxygen delivery to the tissues depends on several components.

   Oxygen delivery = oxygen content × CO

   Oxygen Content = hemoglobin (Hb) × oxygen saturation

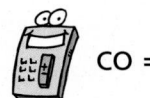   **CO = SV × HR**

Role of Hemoglobin in Oxygen Transport

Hemoglobin concentration is directly related to the amount of oxygen carried in the blood. Oxygen must be bound to hemoglobin for it to be transported by hemoglobin to the tissues. If oxygen is maximally combined with hemoglobin in a 4:1 ratio, it is 100% saturated. One gram of fully saturated hemoglobin carries 1.34 milliliters of oxygen. Desaturation of hemoglobin is most commonly caused by ventilation or perfusion abnormalities or by decreased oxygen tension in the alveoli. Supplemental oxygen is a primary intervention for both problems.

Oxygen Consumption

Oxygen consumption (VO_2) is a measurement of the amount of oxygen consumed and is used as an indicator of oxygen supply. The formula for oxygen consumption uses the oxygen delivery formula, but it also includes the difference between arterial and venous oxygen saturation. Normally, a difference of approximately 5 milliliters per deciliter (ml/dl) exists between oxygen content in the arteries and veins. oxygen consumption is approximately 250 ml/min. A greater portion of oxygen will be extracted from the blood when oxygen supply is insufficient, lowering the oxygen content on the venous side of circulation.

In patients who are critically ill, oxygen demand will dramatically increase. In a patient with a normally functioning cardiovascular system, CO increases above normal to maintain an adequate oxygen supply. However, critically ill patients lose the ability to increase CO (compensation) and may have a CO within normal limits but with an increased oxygen consumption and decreased mixed venous saturation.

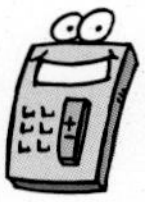

Oxygen consumption (VO_2) = cardiac index (CO ÷ BSA) × 10 × [Hb × 1.34 × (arterial saturation − venous saturation)]

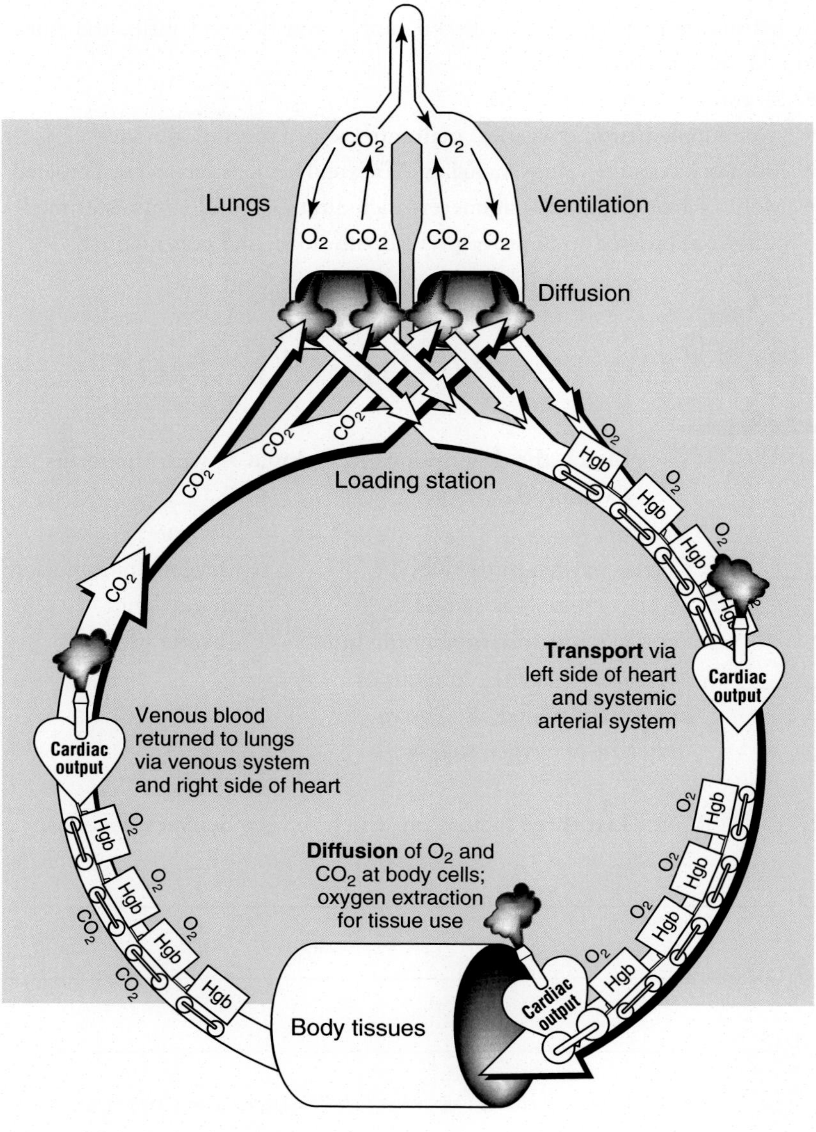

Oxygen delivery is dependent on CO, hemoglobin, and arterial oxygen saturation. CO can be manipulated with the use of fluids or diuretics, vasopressors or vasodilators, and positive or negative inotropic agents.

Critically ill patients should be assessed for adequate CO, BP, and tissue oxygenation by monitoring hemodynamic variables.

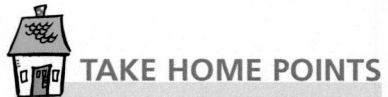

TAKE HOME POINTS

Normal oxygen consumption
   value: 250 ml/min
Range: 180 to 280 ml/min

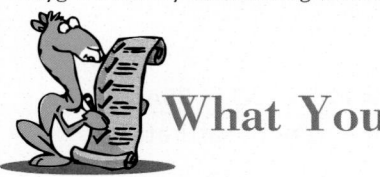

What You DO

In maintaining the patient's oxygen supply and demand ratio, the nurse should provide the following:
- Monitor oxygen saturations.
- Give supplemental oxygen to maintain oxygen saturation above 92%.
- Monitor laboratory values, including ABGs and hemoglobin levels as ordered.
- Monitor hemodynamic parameters including CO, and administer medications as ordered to improve preload, afterload, and contractility.

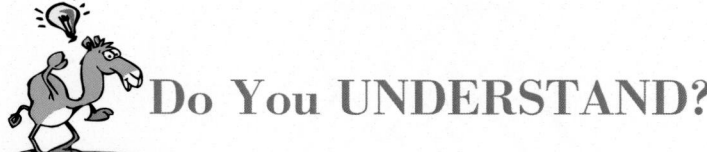

Do You UNDERSTAND?

DIRECTIONS: Match the descriptions in Column A with the terms in Column B.

Column A

_____ 1. Carries oxygen in the blood
_____ 2. Most commonly is caused by
            ventilation/perfusion abnormalities
_____ 3. Measurement of the amount of
            oxygen consumed; used as an
            indicator of oxygen supply

Column B

a. Oxygen consumption
b. Hemoglobin
c. Desaturation

DIRECTIONS: List three factors on which oxygen delivery depends.

4. _____

5. _____

6. _____

Answers: 1. b; 2. c; 3. a; 4. cardiac output; 5. hemoglobin; 6. arterial oxygen saturation.

3 Hemodynamic Monitoring Equipment

Five basic components make up the hemodynamic monitoring system: (1) an indwelling intravascular catheter, (2) a pressure transducer to amplify the signal accurately, (3) a cable to transmit the signal to the monitor, (4) a bedside monitor, and (5) a pressure bag and tubing with a flush device and solution. This chapter discusses the equipment and the setting up, leveling, zeroing, and troubleshooting procedures.

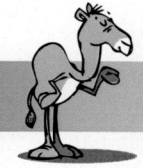

What IS a Pulmonary Artery Catheter?

The type of hemodynamic monitoring needed determines the catheter type and placement. The pulmonary artery (PA) catheter is a flexible, hollow catheter with multiple ports and corresponding lumens. The catheter is 100 centimeters long from the tip. Every 10 centimeters are marked with a black line to allow for estimating the catheter's location upon insertion.

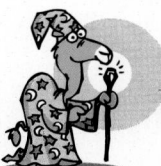

What You NEED TO KNOW

Currently, several types of PA catheters are available with various features and varying numbers of lumens. A PA catheter may have four or five lumens.

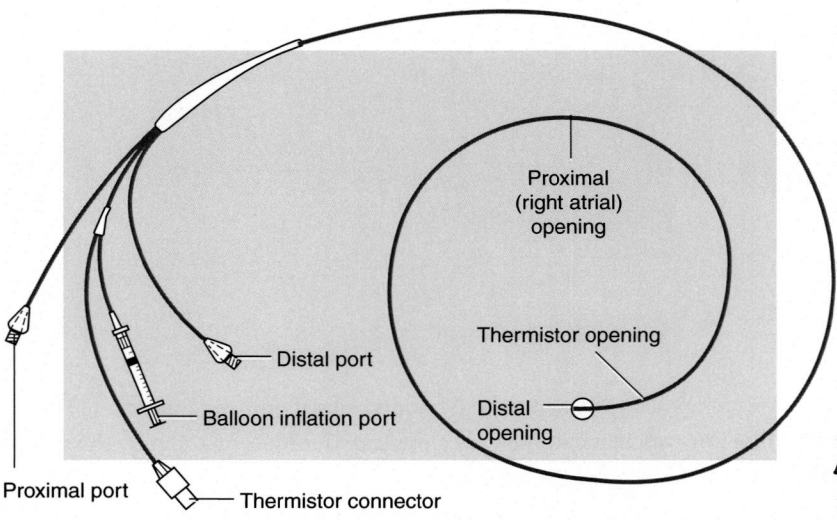

A four-lumen catheter has the following:

1. Proximal injectate port for monitoring right atrial pressures
2. PA distal port for measuring PA systolic, diastolic, and mean pressures
3. Balloon inflation port to allow for inflation of the balloon at the distal tip of the catheter for the purpose of flotation during insertion and obtaining PA occlusion pressures (also known as pulmonary capillary wedge pressures or pulmonary artery occlusion pressure [PAOP/PCWP])
4. Thermistor wire connector used for connecting to a cable for measuring cardiac output (CO) and blood temperature

The five-lumen PA catheter contains an additional lumen called the *proximal infusion port*. The opening to this port is located in the right atrium just proximal to the opening for the right atrial (central venous pressure [CVP]) port.

Other types of PA catheters may contain an additional lumen for the dual purpose of inserting a pacemaker electrode into the right ventricle or fluid infusion. Some catheters are equipped with fiberoptic wires, providing the ability to measure mixed venous oxygen saturation (SVO_2). Other types of catheter provide continuous CO monitoring.

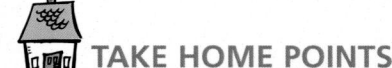

TAKE HOME POINTS

For patients with septal defects, inflate the balloon with carbon dioxide (CO_2). If the balloon ruptures, CO_2 is readily absorbed and minimizes the risk of air embolization.

- **The balloon is inflated with air or CO_2 but NEVER with fluids.**
- **The balloon should be filled with the minimal amount of air or CO_2 required for the process of obtaining the PAOP/PCWP. Catheter manufacturers have recommended guidelines for the maximum amount of air for balloon inflation. NEVER EXCEED the manufacturer's recommendations (usually 1.5 ml air).**
- **Over-inflation may result in balloon rupture or too much pressure on the PA, causing it to rupture. PULMONARY ARTERY RUPTURE IS A MEDICAL EMERGENCY!**

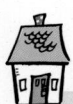

Indications for Pulmonary Artery Catheter Monitoring

The PA catheter helps differentiate causes of fluid status alteration, particularly when the heart or kidneys are not functioning properly. Monitoring PA pressures helps in assessing left ventricular function. It also helps in determining potential causes when right-sided and left-sided pressures do not correlate with expected values.

Pressures Monitored with a Pulmonary Artery Catheter

PA catheters allow for monitoring the PA systolic, diastolic, and mean pressures. The catheter can also monitor right atrial pressure (CVP) and PCWP (also called PAOP, which reflects left ventricular end–diastolic pressure). In addition, CO, vascular resistance (systemic and pulmonary), and mixed SVO$_2$ can be monitored.

CVP measurements can be directly measured by several different methods. If a PA catheter is inserted, the right atrial port (proximal injectate port) can be used for monitoring right atrial pressures (CVP). Another method of measuring CVP is by placing a central line in the inferior vena cava, superior vena cava, or right atrium. When using a central venous catheter to measure pressures, the distal port must be used, which more closely approximates the location of the CVP lumen of the PA catheter.

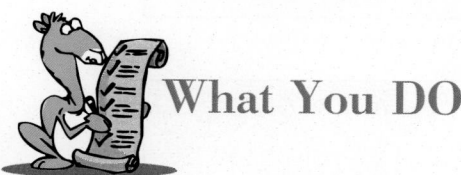

What You DO

Catheter Insertion

The physician, using sterile technique, inserts the PA catheter. The PA catheter can be percutaneously inserted or by a cutdown approach. Waveform analysis can identify catheter location; therefore fluoroscopy is not usually used.

Hemodynamic pressures are affected by the position of the catheter tip and blood flow. Appropriate catheter length and position are essential in producing waveforms representative of the patient's pressures.

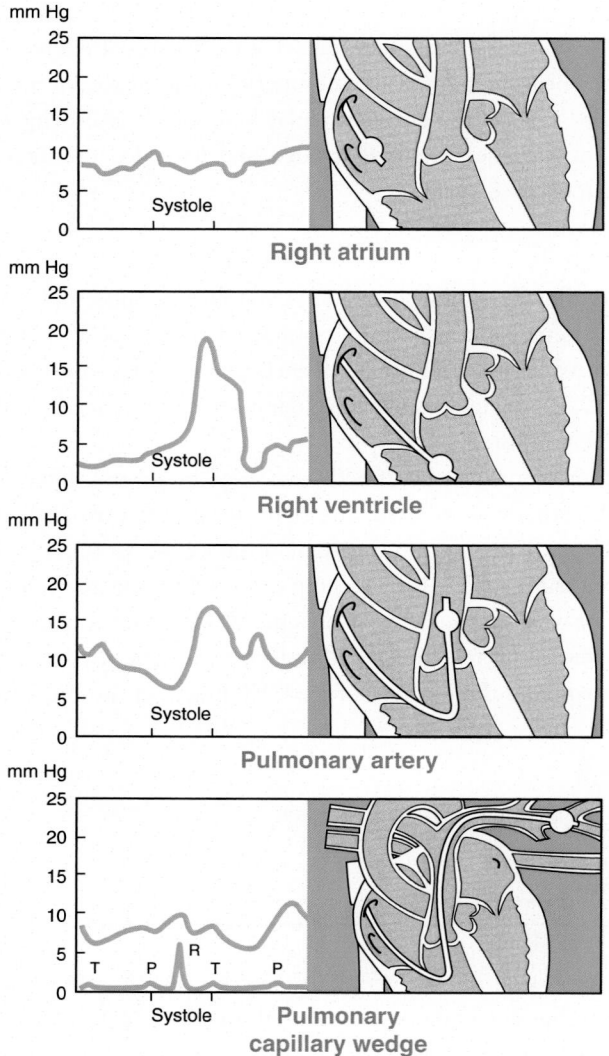

Once inserted, the catheter is progressed and the balloon is inflated, causing the catheter to drift with the flow of blood from the right atrium to the right ventricle through the pulmonic valve into the PA. When the catheter is inserted without fluoroscopy, observing the waveform identifies the location of the catheter.

The most common insertion sites include one of the following veins: sub-clavian, internal jugular, femoral, and sometimes brachial.

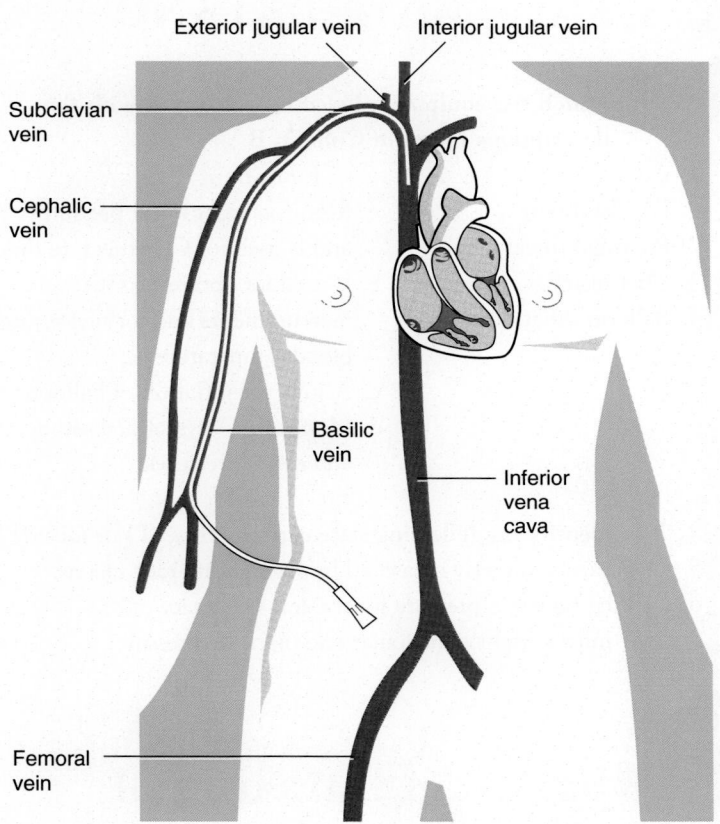

Exterior jugular vein   Interior jugular vein

Subclavian vein

Cephalic vein

Basilic vein

Inferior vena cava

Femoral vein

Potential complications of a PA catheter may include ventricular ectopy, PA infarction or rupture, air emboli, infection, and sepsis.

Pulmonary hypertension and advanced age are factors that can predispose a patient to PA rupture when a PA catheter is placed.

Catheter or Equipment-Related Problems

Because PA catheters are inserted into the venous system and are directed with the flow of blood, catheter whip (catheter noise or catheter fling) can occur. This movement of the catheter during the contraction of the right ventricle causes an artifact to be superimposed on the waveform. Adding a high-frequency filter to the monitoring system can eliminate catheter whip. If no filter is used, correct and consistent waveform measurement is imperative. Refer to institutional policy for frequency and protocols regarding waveform measurement.

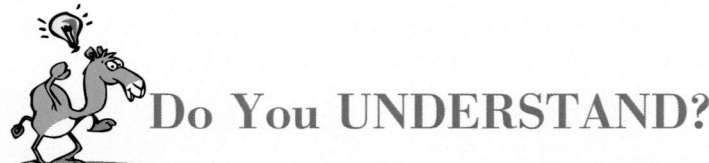

Do You UNDERSTAND?

DIRECTIONS: **Match the equipment listed in Column A with the descriptions found in Column B.**

Column A

_____ 1. PA distal port

_____ 2. Proximal injectate port

_____ 3. Thermistor

_____ 4. Balloon inflation port

Column B

a. Monitors right atrial pressures and is used for CO injectate fluid.

b. Is used for obtaining CO measurements and for measuring blood temperature.

c. Allows for inflation of balloon.

d. Monitors PA systolic, diastolic, and mean pressures.

DIRECTIONS: **Identify the following statements as *true* (T) or *false* (F).**

_____ 5. CVP can be directly measured by several different means.

_____ 6. CVP is the mean pressure for the left ventricle.

_____ 7. CVP reflects right ventricular end diastolic pressure.

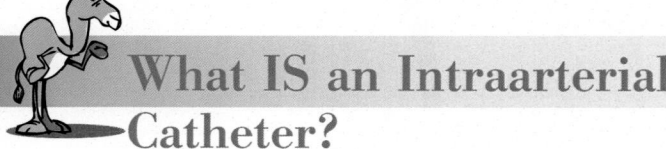

What IS an Intraarterial Catheter?

An intraarterial catheter is a short catheter (usually less than 4 inches) that is commonly inserted into the radial artery, although other insertion sites such as the brachial, femoral, axillary, or pedal arteries may be used.

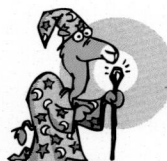

What You NEED TO KNOW

Invasive arterial monitoring allows for the direct measurement of systolic, diastolic, and mean BP levels. Direct BP monitoring is considered more accurate than indirect noninvasive monitoring, especially during conditions

Answers: 1. d; 2. a; 3. b; 4. c; 5. T; 6. F; 7. T.

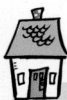

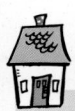
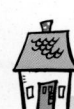

of altered peripheral resistance, abnormal body temperature, or abnormal blood flow. (For further information on arterial pressure monitoring and waveforms, refer to Chapter 4.)

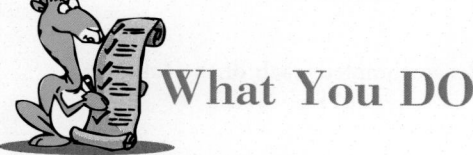

What You DO

The nurse should:

• Gather the equipment for arterial line insertion per institutional protocol.

• Set up the pressure tubing and transducer system, and fill the pressure bag with fluid, inflating it with 300 millimeters mercury (300 mm Hg).

• Turn on the monitoring system before inserting the catheter.

• Assist the physician with insertion per institutional protocols using sterile technique.

• Once the catheter is inserted, attach the catheter to the high-pressure tubing of the transducer system.

• Set the scales on the monitor to a range higher than the anticipated pressure to ensure the arterial waveform will be the appropriate size to reflect accurate arterial pressures (usually in the 0 to 200 range). The scale range must be greater than the arterial pressures, or the waveforms will be dampened and may lead to inappropriate treatments.

• Follow the procedure for leveling and zeroing the system (refer to the section on leveling or zeroing later in this chapter).

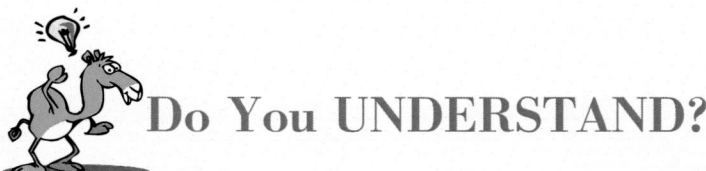

Do You UNDERSTAND?

DIRECTIONS: **Fill in the blanks to complete each of the following**
                statements.

1. The six basic components of a hemodynamic monitoring system are

   _____

   _____

   _____

   _____

   _____

   _____

2. A PA catheter helps differentiate causes of

   _____

   _____.

3. PA catheters allow for monitoring of the PA _____,

   _____, and _____ pressures.

4. A PA PCWP/PAOP reflects _____ _____

   _____–_____ _____.

5. PA catheters _____ _____ allow for BP monitoring.

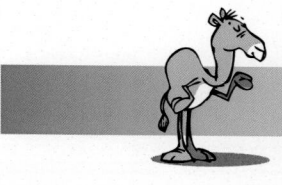

What IS the Equipment Needed for Hemodynamic Monitoring?

The equipment required for hemodynamic monitoring includes the catheter, tubing, transducer, cable, and monitor. The catheter, tubing, and transducer system should be as direct and short as possible. The pressure tubing from the catheter to the transducer should be stiff and noncompliant to reflect accurate pressures from the patient. Any air bubbles should be evacuated from the tubing during setup. Stopcocks and tubing connections should be initially tightened and monitored for loose connections or fluid leaks.

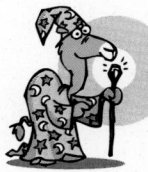

What You NEED TO KNOW

Transducers are devices that measure pressure, flow, temperature, light intensity, and sound. The transducer converts the physiologic event into an electrical waveform. This waveform is transmitted to the monitor through a cable.

A bedside monitor is an instrument used to display and record the physiologic events. Most frequently, bedside monitors reflect hemodynamic pressures as a waveform and a digital display.

Any invasive intravascular monitoring catheter should be attached to a system that has a flush solution (usually either heparinized or nonheparinized normal saline) under pressure through an inflatable pressure bag. The system should also have rigid, noncompliant pressure tubing with a transducer and flush device that controls the flow of solution through the system.

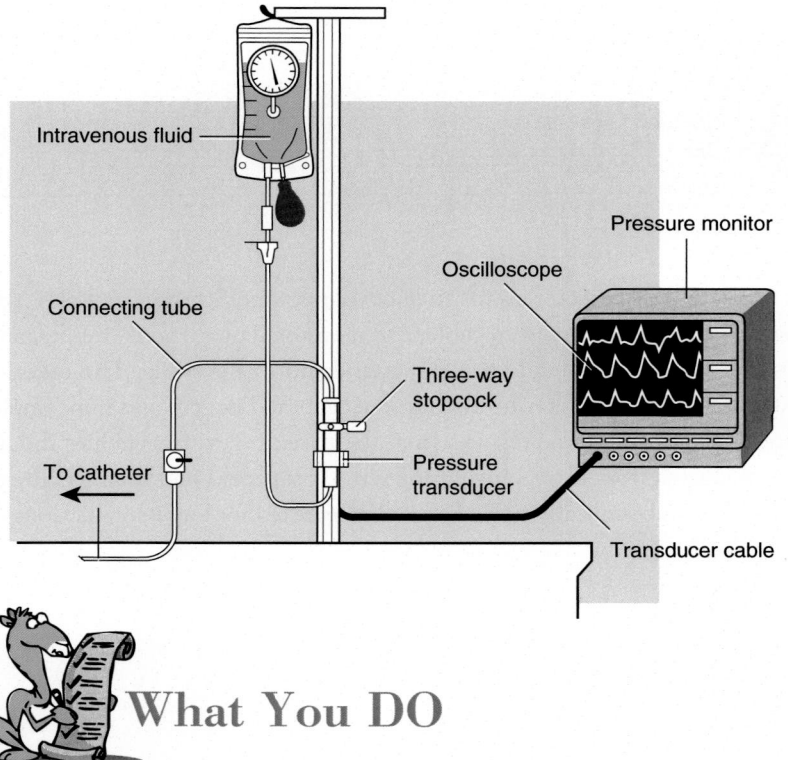

Intravenous fluid

Connecting tube

To catheter

Oscilloscope

Pressure monitor

Three-way stopcock

Pressure transducer

Transducer cable

What You DO

The transducer used for monitoring pressures must be leveled and zero referenced to obtain reliable measurements. This setup standardizes the equipment. To level a transducer, position the air-fluid interface (the stopcock at the top of the transducer) at the level of the patient's right atrium. This position is referred to as the *phlebostatic axis* and is located at the fourth intercostal space, midaxillary position.

Leveling the Transducer

Once the equipment is assembled and the monitor is turned on, the transducer needs to be leveled. Leveling the transducer is the process of referencing the tip of the intravascular catheter horizontally to a specific position on the transducer, usually at the top or side stopcock of the transducer. This leveling allows the transducer to be opened to air to a zero-reference position. When the transducer is mounted on a pole in a transducer holder, the transducer holder can be adjusted to ensure that the stopcock height is level with the tip of the intravascular catheter, usually at the phlebostatic axis. Leveling can be accomplished with a carpenter's level. Leveling should be repeated when the position of the patient or the height of the bed is altered.

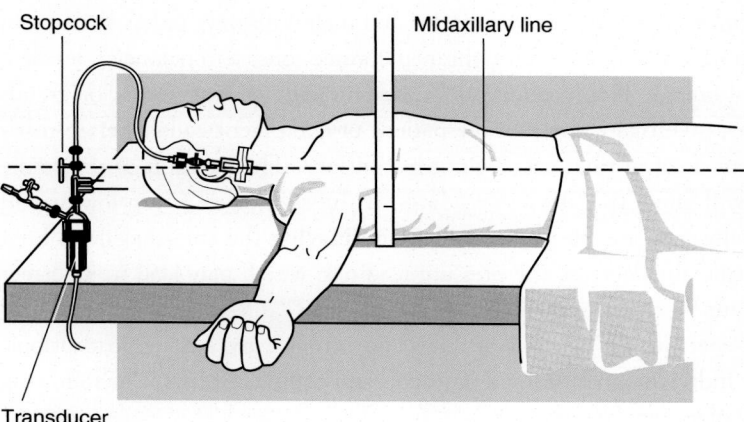

Stopcock
Midaxillary line
Transducer

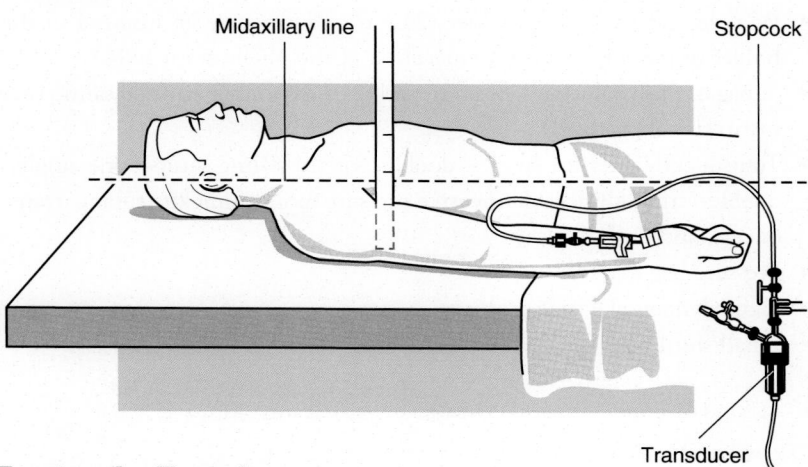

Midaxillary line
Stopcock
Transducer

TAKE HOME POINTS

Often the transducer is placed in a transducer holder attached to an IV pole; however, it can be taped directly to the patient's chest or arm. When the transducer is taped to the patient, it is not necessary to rezero with position changes; however, check institutional policies regarding indications for rezeroing. It is helpful to use a level for ensuring the appropriate height of the transducer when mounted on an IV pole.

Zeroing the Transducer

Distortion in the transducer must be compensated for electronically. This process is referred to as "zeroing the transducer." The process of zeroing should be performed after the catheter is initially inserted but before the first pressure measurements are obtained. Institutional protocols regarding frequency of zeroing should be followed. However, the transducer should be zeroed after any intervention that alters the patient's position, after any repositioning of the patient, or at least once during a shift. To zero the transducer, the nurse should:

- Open the stopcock on the transducer to air and close it to the patient.
- Depress the automatic zero button on the monitor. The digital readout on the monitor should display "0."
- Close the stopcock to air and open to the patient once the zero reference is obtained.
- Fast flush the system.

Do not rely on pressure waveforms and digital displays unless the system is accurately assembled with tightened connections, zero balanced, leveled, and calibrated. If any question of inaccuracies of waveforms or trends remains, investigate any possible patient or equipment causes before instituting medical or pharmacologic interventions. The position of the transducer will affect the pressure readings. If the transducer is too low, it will artificially increase the pressure readings. Having the transducer too high will artificially decrease the pressure readings, which may lead to incorrect treatment for the patient.

The specifics of PA and arterial line setups vary among institutions. Follow individual institutional protocols and equipment lists. The following is a list of *potential* equipment:

- IV pole and transducer holder (The transducer may be inserted in the holder or placed on the patient's chest at the phlebostatic axis.)
- A bag of flush solution—often heparinized or nonheparinized saline (per institutional protocol)
- Transducer cables for single-, double-, or triple-line setup—one single-, double-, triple-disposable invasive pressure monitoring kit (tubing, transducers, and flush device)
- Pressure bag
- Hemodynamic bedside monitor
- Small sterile cup or bowl of sterile saline to test balloon integrity

Preparation for Hemodynamic Monitoring

The nurse should:

- Gather the equipment for line setup and PA catheter insertion per institutional protocols.
- Turn on monitoring system before catheter insertion.
- Explain the procedure to the patient.
- Ensure all consent forms are signed.
- Have emergency equipment available.
- Attach the transducer holder to the pole.
- Slide all transducers into the holder.
- Tighten connections along pressure tubing.
- Spike bag of flush solution (heparinized or nonheparinized saline) with IV spike portion of pressure tubing set, and insert flush solution into pressure bag.
- Flush each pressure line (PA, CVP, and arterial line [ART]) to tip of pressure tubing and to each stopcock port.

> **Do not rely on pressure waveforms and digital displays unless the system is accurately assembled with tightened connections, zero balanced, leveled, and calibrated.**

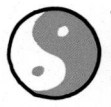 While preparing the patient, consider any cultural or religious beliefs that may influence the patient's understanding and attitudes about the procedure.

- Apply 300 mm Hg pressure to pressure bag.
- Inspect tubing, transducers, and stopcocks for air bubbles and remove any if present.
- Replace any vented caps on stopcocks with nonvented (dead-end) caps.
- Recap distal end of pressure tubing until ready to connect to catheter and patient.
- Ensure transducer cable is connected to monitor.
- Set the scales on the monitor to the 0 to 40 range to reflect pressures accurately.
- Follow the procedure for leveling and zeroing the system.

Preparation for Catheter Insertion

The nurse should:
- Prepare a sterile field.
- Open catheter and provide catheter insertion tray and suturing equipment (if not included in tray) using sterile technique.
- Depending on the contents of the catheter insertion tray, gather additional 4 × 4 gauze pads, sterile towels, and a sterile gown.
- Obtain syringes with 10 ml of saline flush solution (may be heparinized or nonheparinized, depending on institutional policy).
- Test the balloon before inserting a PA catheter. Inflate the balloon port with 1.0 to 1.5 ml air. Using sterile technique, place the inflated balloon in a sterile bowl filled with sterile water, observe for any air leakage (bubbles), and then allow the balloon to deflate.
- Flush all ports along with any attached stopcocks, using sterile technique. Follow institutional protocols and physician preference for flushing the catheter before insertion.
- Slide sleeve protector over catheter if used.
- Cover prepared tray with sterile towels.

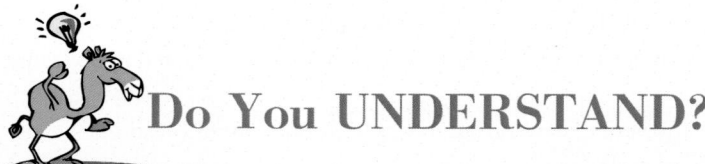

Do You UNDERSTAND?

DIRECTIONS: Match the descriptions in Column A to the terms listed in Column B.

Column A

_____ 1. Converts a physiologic event into an electronic display

_____ 2. Displays and records events

_____ 3. Is essential for obtaining reliable measurements

_____ 4. Is the fourth intercostal space; midaxillary line

Column B

a. Phlebostatic axis

b. Transducer

c. Monitor

d. Leveling and zeroing

e. PA catheter

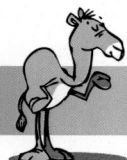

What IS a Square Wave Test?

The *square wave test* is a procedure used to test the dynamic response of the fluid-filled monitoring system to reproduce the patient's pressure accurately on the monitor. This calibration is performed on all hemodynamic systems before assuming that the pressures and waveforms are accurate.

 Visit the Edwards Lifesciences web site: www.edwards.com **and** the Pulmonary Catheter Education Project web site: www. pacep.com **for additional information on understanding hemodynamic monitoring.**

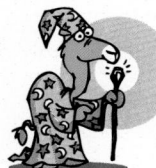

What You NEED TO KNOW

Dynamic response testing (the square wave test) can identify whether the system accurately reflects the pressures and waveforms from the patient. An optimal system produces an accurate square wave test, which consists of one to two oscillations and then a return to a normal waveform. If the system has extraneous resistance, the upstroke of the square wave will slur and less than one to two oscillations will be observed before returning to the patient's waveform. This represents an overdamped system, which will cause the patient's waveform to display a falsely decreased systolic pressure.

Answers: 1. b; 2. c; 3. d; 4. a.

Square wave test configuration

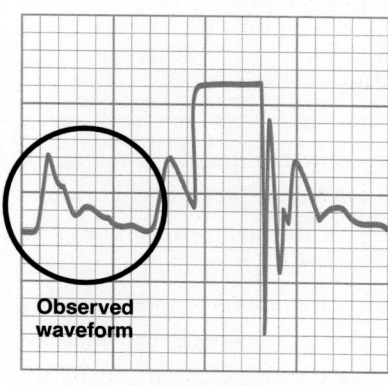

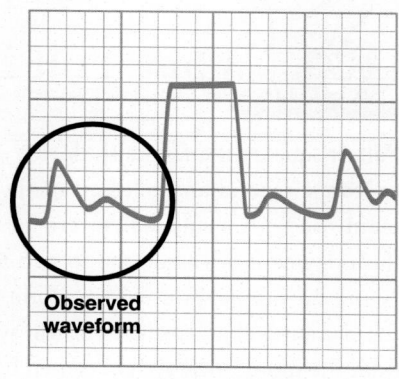

Accurate square wave test

Overdamped system

In addition, the waveform tracing may be diminished with poorly defined components. If the waveform tracing has extra oscillations (more than two) before returning to the baseline after the fast flush, the monitor may falsely display elevated systolic pressures and potentially low diastolic pressures, which is referred to as an underdamped system.

Square wave test configuration

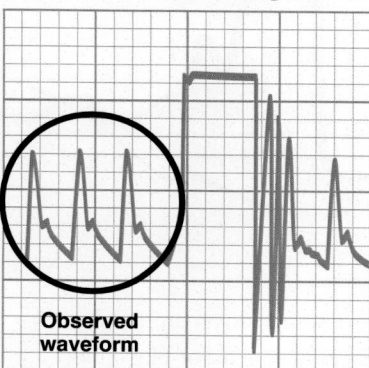

Underdamped system

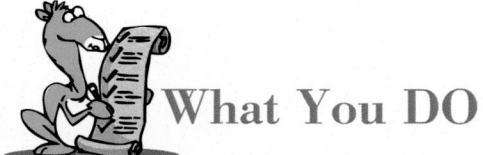

What You DO

Pull or squeeze the fast flush device connected to the transducer tubing for at least 1 second and release rapidly. The waveform tracing should have a rapid rise with a squared pattern to the top of the graph paper. Once the flush device is released, one to two narrow oscillations should be observed before the normal pressure waveform returns. This procedure shows whether the damping characteristics of the system (loss of the energy or vibrations from the monitoring system caused by internal resistance) accurately reflect digital readouts and pressure waveforms. The square wave test should be repeated when waveform accuracy is in question.

Interventions for Overdamping or Underdamping

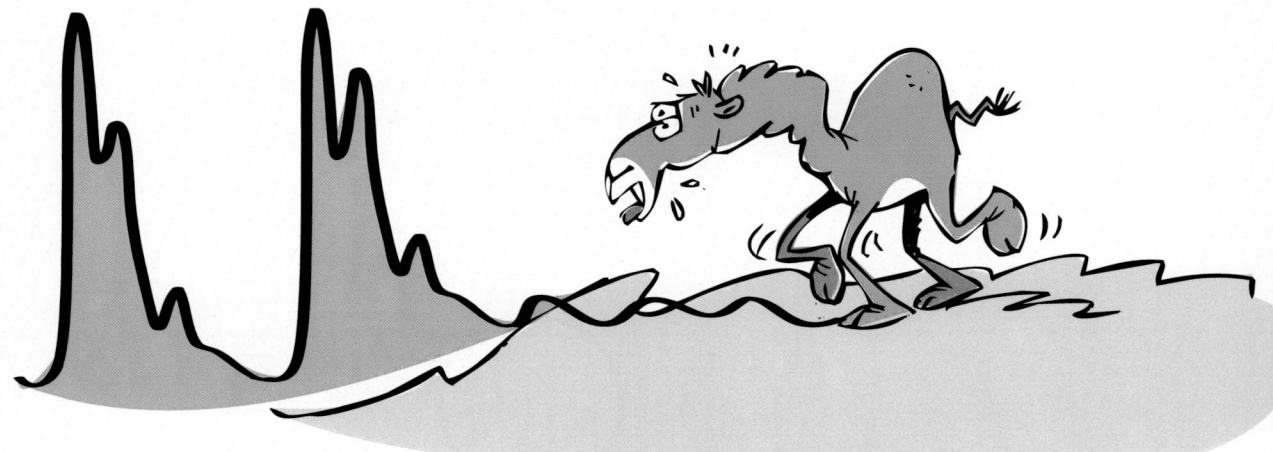

Interventions for an overdamped system include:
- Checking the tubing and system for blood clots, air bubbles, or blood left in the tubing after blood sampling.
- Ensuring that the tubing from the transducer to the patient is rigid and as short as possible and that all connections are secure.
- Ensuring that no kinks in the tubing can be found.

Interventions for an underdamped system include ensuring that all air bubbles (including pinpoint bubbles) have been removed from the system and that large bore, short tubing is being used.

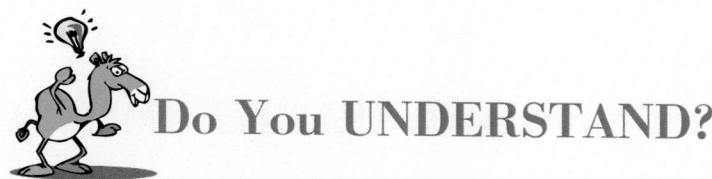

Do You UNDERSTAND?

DIRECTIONS: Identify the following statements as *true* (T) or *false* (F).

_____ 1. The square wave test can identify whether the system accurately reflects the pressures and waveforms from the patient.

_____ 2. Slurring of the upstroke of the square wave represents underdamping.

_____ 3. An underdamped system can falsely elevate systolic pressures.

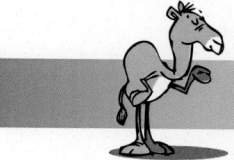

What IS the Importance of Patient Positioning?

Correct patient positioning is important in obtaining accurate pressure measurements. Patients are often placed in a supine position; however, situations exist in which the patient is unable to tolerate lying flat. If the hemodynamic system has been properly leveled and zeroed, then the patient may be placed in a backrest position of 0 to 60 degrees without a significant change in the PA pressure or wedge pressure measurements.

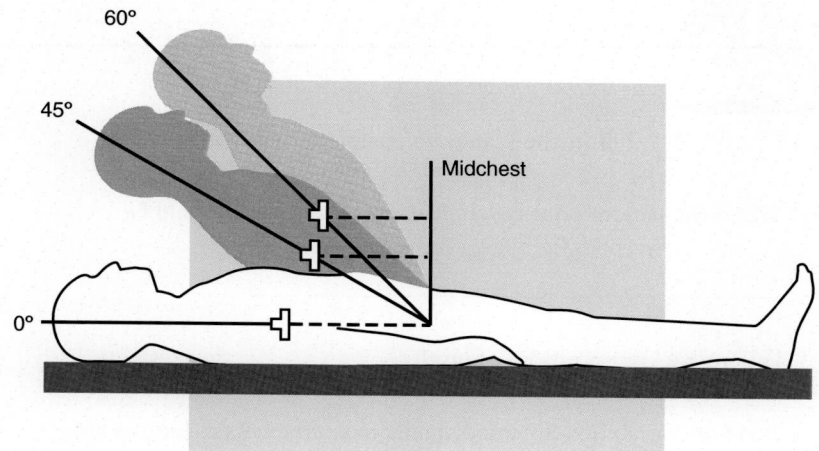

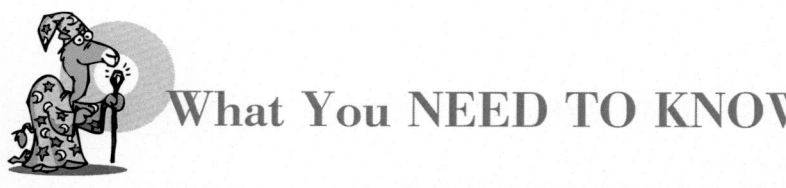

What You NEED TO KNOW

When position changes are made, the transducer should be leveled and the change in position documented on the hemodynamic flow sheet. For accuracy, once position changes are made, allow 5 minutes before obtaining pressure measurements. Consistency is the important factor in positioning.

Patient positioning for measuring pressures has been the subject of many research studies that support the belief that backrest positions up to 60 degrees have little effect on the variability of hemodynamic measurements as long as the phlebostatic axis and appropriate leveling have been accomplished.

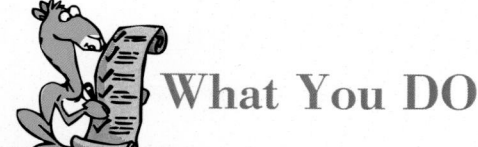

What You DO

When monitoring right atrial pressures, the nurse should ensure the patient is supine and flat or with the head of the bed elevated up to 60 degrees. Research has shown that measures taken with a patient in a sidelying position may reflect distorted values because of a change in intrathoracic pressures. The best position is supine and within the 0 to 60 degree range.

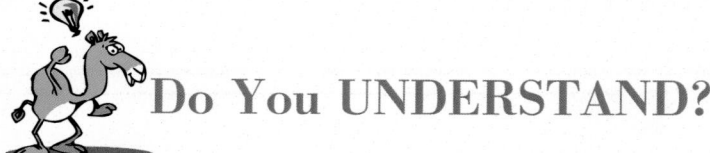

Do You UNDERSTAND?

DIRECTIONS: **Fill in the blanks to complete each statement.**

1. When the patient position changes, the transducer should be

   _____.

2. Patient backrest positions of up to _____ degrees have little

   effect on variability of hemodynamic measurements as long as the

   _____ _____ and leveling has been established.

Answers: 1. leveled; 2. 60, phlebostatic axis.

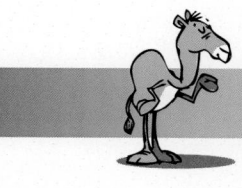

What IS the Importance of Identifying Monitoring Problems?

Pressure measurements and waveforms should correlate with the patient's clinical picture. Technical problems with the monitoring system may result in distorted waveforms, inaccurate pressure measurements, or inability to obtain a waveform and pressure. Many therapeutic treatments are based on the values obtained with the PA catheter. If there is a systemic problem, then inappropriate treatments may be initiated with potentially deleterious effects to the patient.

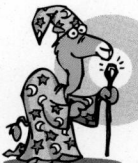

What You NEED TO KNOW

Troubleshooting potential monitoring problems includes following the system from the patient to the monitor.

- Ensure correct, consistent patient positioning, a leveled transducer that has been rezeroed, and an intact tubing and a flush system without air bubbles or loose connections.
- Check the pressure bag for adequate inflation pressure.

If no visible clues are observed in the tubing system, consider the potential for problems within the catheter or related to catheter position. (Refer to Chapter 6, Pulmonary Artery Pressure Monitoring.)

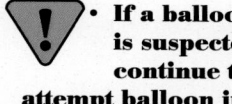

- **If a balloon rupture is suspected, NEVER continue to attempt balloon inflation. Label the balloon port as unusable and notify the physician. Follow institutional and unit protocols for further interventions.**
- **Spontaneous catheter wedging can result in PA necrosis or rupture! Following institutional protocol, slowly withdraw the catheter until a normal PA waveform appears. A catheter should only be wedged for two to three respiratory cycles to avoid damage to the vessel. If a wedge waveform is observed, it is urgent that this be corrected immediately.**
- **NEVER forcibly irrigate the catheter! This may dislodge the obstructing clot and result in embolization.**

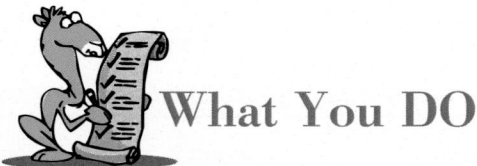

What You DO

Troubleshooting System Problems

PROBLEM	POTENTIAL CAUSES	SOLUTIONS
Inability to obtain a PCWP or PAOP	Balloon has ruptured. Catheter has migrated backward.	Observe waveform for confirmation of catheter position. Notify physician. Obtain a chest x-ray (per protocol) to confirm catheter position. Follow institutional protocols and policy.
Dampened PA waveform	Air is observed in the tubing. Blood has clotted within the catheter or at the tip. Catheter has kinks or knots. Loose tubing connections are observed. Catheter has spontaneously migrated forward. Inappropriate monitor scales have been selected (i.e., if a PA pressure is measured using arterial pressure scale, then the waveform would be dampened). Transducer is cracked.	Inspect tubing for air or blood. Air in system should be evacuated before reaching catheter. Ensure pressure bag is fully inflated. Obtain a chest x-ray (per protocol). Ensure connections are tightened. **This is an emergency!** Notify physician immediately, and follow institutional protocol for catheter pull back. Change monitor scales to the appropriate setting for hemodynamic value being monitored. Inspect transducer, change entire transducer system.
No waveform	Transducer is defective. Monitor or system has been incorrectly set up. Stopcocks are turned "off" to the patient. Monitor is turned "off." Pressure cable is defective. Catheter tip is clotted.	Change transducer system. Check system from patient to monitor, ensure correct cable connection, correct line set up, appropriate scales. Check stopcock, turn "on" to the patient and transducer; turn "off" to side port. Check "on/off" switch. Change cables. Notify physician. Clotted catheter requires catheter replacement.

PAOP, Pulmonary artery occlusion pressure; *PCWP,* pulmonary capillary wedge pressure.

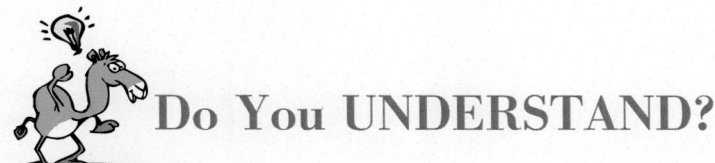

Do You UNDERSTAND?

DIRECTIONS: List three potential system problems that may be encountered with PA monitoring.

1. _____

2. _____

3. _____

Answers: 1. inability to obtain a PCWP or PAOP; 2. dampened PA waveform; 3. no waveform.

CHAPTER

4 Arterial Pressure Monitoring

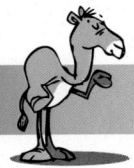

What IS Arterial Pressure Monitoring?

Arterial pressure monitoring is an accurate, direct, and invasive method to measure and monitor a patient's blood pressure (BP). This method of measuring BP allows for continuous BP readings through a catheter inserted directly into an artery. By providing an accurate and continuous BP reading, a critical care nurse is able to assess and manage the patient more efficiently.

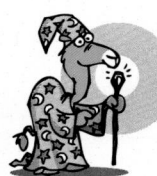

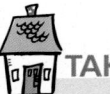

TAKE HOME POINTS

- Noninvasive (indirect) BP readings should be periodically obtained to determine the correlation between the cuff and arterial line BP levels.
- A patient may have blood drawn from an arterial catheter inserted for continuous BP monitoring. Blood draws from an arterial catheter save time and, when performed properly, are painless for the patient.

What You NEED TO KNOW

Arterial pressure monitoring is one of the most commonly used hemodynamic monitoring techniques in the critical care setting. Most patients admitted to a critical care unit will have an arterial catheter inserted to assist in monitoring sudden changes in BP. This continuous monitoring allows for rapid interventions. It also allows for frequent blood sampling and serial blood gas measurement. Those who benefit from arterial pressure monitoring include patients who:

- Are hypotensive
- Are hypertensive
- Are receiving vasoactive medications (Arterial pressure monitoring in patients having vasoactive medications titrated allows for immediate feedback on the patient's response to the treatment.)

⚠ • **For very unstable patients, direct arterial line BP monitoring is preferred because it is the most accurate.**
• **Inserting an arterial catheter may be contra-indicated in patients who have received a thrombo-lytic agent as a result of their increased bleeding potential. Therefore if an arterial line is being considered in this patient group, it should be inserted before administering any thrombolytic agents.**

⚠ **Make certain all con-nections on the sys-tem are tight and not leaking. Any loose connec-tions can lead to a rapid and massive loss of blood.**

• Are undergoing or recovering from major surgeries including vascular, thoracic, abdominal, or neurologic procedures
• Require frequent arterial blood gas monitoring

Once the patient has been identified as a candidate for arterial pressure monitoring, the nurse will need to collect the following appropriate equipment and supplies:
• Catheter
• Pressurized fluid system (flush bag, pressure tubing, and pressure device)
• Transducer
• Monitoring cable
• Monitor

(For further information regarding the setup and initiation of hemodynamic monitoring, see Chapter 3.)

A physician usually places an arterial catheter, but sometimes other qualified health care professionals may insert an arterial catheter. Be sure to check institutional policy and procedures.

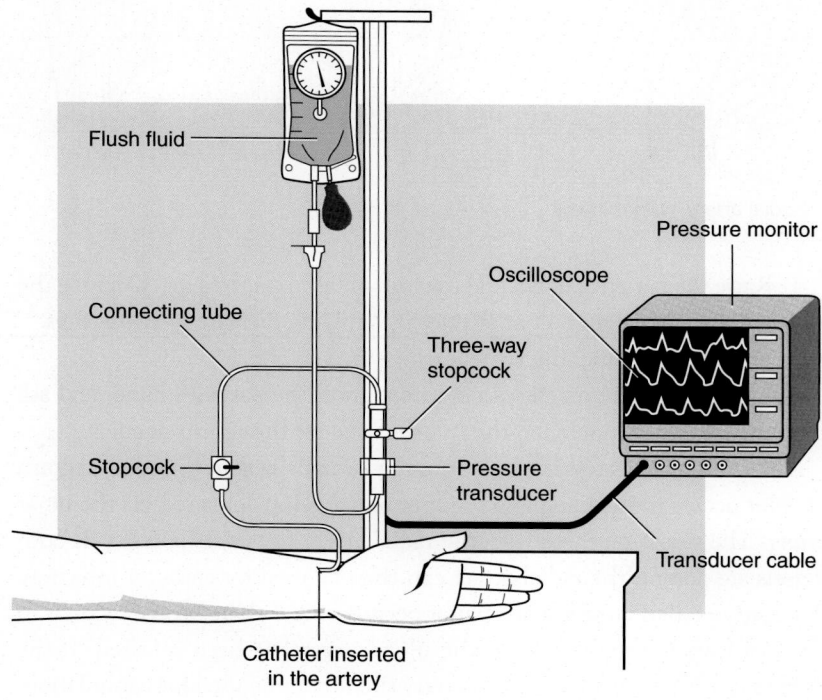

Flush fluid

Connecting tube

Stopcock

Three-way stopcock

Pressure transducer

Oscilloscope

Pressure monitor

Transducer cable

Catheter inserted in the artery

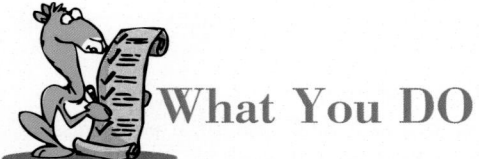

What You DO

The arterial catheter is a short catheter inserted into an accessible artery such as the radial, brachial, axillary, femoral, or pedal. The most often used site is the radial artery, unless the radial pulse is not palpable. Before inserting a catheter into the radial artery, it is important to determine ulnar artery patency. Determining ulnar artery patency assists in concluding whether blood flow from the radial artery is obstructed. If obstructed, collateral blood will then flow into the hand via the ulnar artery. Ulnar artery patency is easy to assess by performing the Allen's test. The Allen's test is made up of three steps:

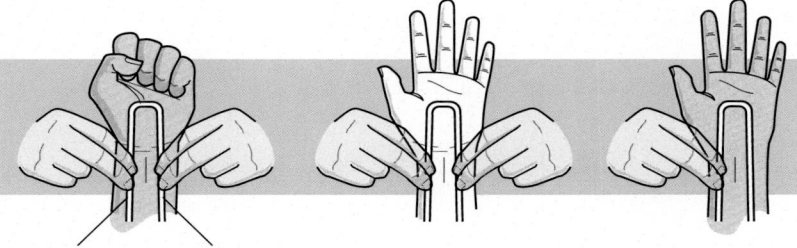

Radial artery   Ulnar artery

1. Raise the patient's hand, and ask him or her to make a fist. Occlude the patient's radial and ulnar arteries by applying pressure over the sites.
2. Observe for blanching (paleness).
3. Release pressure on the ulnar artery, lower the patient's hand, and ask the patient to unclench the fist. Observe for the return of color.

A positive Allen's test is when a prompt (usually within 6 seconds) return of color occurs in the hand as a result of blood being delivered via the ulnar artery. The test is repeated with the radial artery to test its patency. If both vessels are patent, the radial artery can then be used for catheter insertion. A negative Allen's test is when pallor persists longer than 5 to 10 seconds in the hand after the pressure on the ulnar artery has been released. If the Allen's test is negative, the radial artery should not be used for cannulation.

Numerous advantages and disadvantages are considered when determining the arterial site of choice for inserting an arterial catheter.

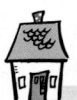

TAKE HOME POINTS

- The radial artery is the most common site used for arterial pressure monitoring.
- An Allen's test should be performed whenever a radial arterial catheter is to be inserted or an arterial puncture is performed to ensure that the blood supply to the hand is not compromised if the radial artery becomes occluded by a thrombus, vascular spasm, or catheter.
- Select the nondominant hand whenever possible to allow the patient to use the more dexterous hand and to minimize the risk of severe permanent disability in the event distal ischemia occurs.

Selecting the Arterial Site for Inserting an Arterial Catheter

ARTERIAL SITE	ADVANTAGES	DISADVANTAGES
Radial	• Easy to access • Easy to identify • Easier to insert catheter when compared with other sites • Easy to assess and document distal circulation • Low distal vascular insufficiency • Minimal immobilization of site • More comfortable than other sites	• Possible nerve injury from insertion trauma or hematoma formation • Small-gauge catheter causing predisposition to overshoot artifact • Thrombus formation high with prolonged use
Brachial	• Large artery • Easy to insert • Low distal vascular insufficiency	• Immobilization of site to attain reading • Uncomfortable site for patient • Possible median nerve injury from insertion trauma or hematoma formation • Possible thrombus formation leading to compromised blood flow to the radial and ulnar arteries
Axillary	• Useful when unable to palpate peripheral pulses • Decreased complications with prolonged use • Less likelihood of overshoot artifact when compared with other sites • Useful site in patients with severe peripheral vascular disease • Low distal vascular insufficiency	• Predisposition to neurologic complications when hematoma is present • Difficult insertion • Possible cerebral air or clot embolism during blood sampling or flushing of the system

Selecting the Arterial Site for Inserting an Arterial Catheter—cont'd

SITE	ADVANTAGES	DISADVANTAGES
Femoral	• Easy to access • Useful when unable to palpate peripheral pulses • Decreased complications with prolonged use	• Immobilized site to attain reading • Catheter insertion may be difficult in presence of atherosclerotic plaques that may embolize • Massive, retroperitoneal hemorrhage is possible
Pedal	• Useful when access to other sites is unavailable	• Causes predisposition to thrombotic occlusion • Difficult insertion because of small size of artery • Immobilized site to attain reading • Uncomfortable site for patient • Patient unable to walk or stand until catheter is discontinued • Site causes predisposition to artifacts and erroneous readings

Before inserting an arterial catheter, the nurse should obtain informed consent. Once the catheter has been inserted and hooked to the pressurized system, the nurse should:

- Place a dressing over the site and change the dressing as warranted or according to institutional policy and procedures.
- Immobilize the joint or limb in a neutral position to prevent kinking or dislodgement of the catheter. Do not hyperextend the wrist; doing so may result in neuromuscular injury to the hand.
- Assess the circulation status of the extremity in which the arterial catheter has been inserted. This assessment should be made every hour and include skin color, temperature, capillary refill, distal pulses (if appropriate), motor function, and sensation.
- Change the flush bag and tubing every 96 hours or according to institutional policy and procedures.
- After discontinuing and removing the arterial catheter, apply and maintain firm, direct pressure for 5 to 10 minutes to ensure adequate clot for-

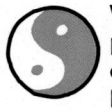

While preparing the patient, consider any cultural or religious beliefs that may influence the patient's understanding and attitudes about the procedure.

• Radial artery catheters in place longer than 48 hours have an increased risk of developing infection and forming a thrombus.
• Arterial line occlusion as a result of the formation of a thrombus will result in ischemia; if not recognized, this ischemia could cause the loss of the affected limb. Follow institutional protocols and policies for management of arterial line occlusions.
• Overaggressive and vigorous flushing of the line may result in air bubbles (air embolism) entering in the direction of blood flow and reaching the aorta, where it could enter the cerebral, systemic, or coronary artery circulation and cause ischemia.
• DO NOT USE ARTERIAL LINES for administering medications. Accidental injection of a medication into the arterial line may result in serious complications such as ischemia or necrosis of the involved

mation over the puncture site. Patients with coagulopathies may require a longer time of firm, direct pressure.

Complications that might occur from catheterization and arterial pressure monitoring include infection, hemorrhage, development of a clot on the tip of the catheter, embolism (clot or air), and decreased distal blood flow to the extremity involved. (For further information regarding possible complications with hemodynamic monitoring, see Chapter 3.)

Do You UNDERSTAND?

DIRECTIONS: Select the correct italicized phrase or phrases within the parentheses to complete each of the following statements.

1. _____ BP readings should be

obtained periodically to determine the correlation between the cuff

and arterial line BPs. (*direct; indirect*)

2. Arterial catheters _____.
(*monitor sudden changes in BP; allow frequent blood sampling; are used to administer medications*)

3. The arterial catheter is a short catheter most often inserted into the

_____ artery.
(*radial; axillary; pedal*)

4. If the Allen's test is _____, the

radial artery should not be used for cannulation. (*positive; negative*)

5. Complications that may occur from catheterization and arterial pres-

Answers: 1. Indirect; 2. monitor sudden changes in BP, allow frequent blood sampling; 3. radial; 4. negative.

sure monitoring include _____.
*(infection and hemorrhage; increased distal blood flow to the involved
extremity)*

What IS an Arterial Pressure Waveform?

An arterial pressure waveform will be displayed once the arterial catheter is
inserted and connected to the pressurized fluid system, transducer, and monitor. The arterial pressure waveform is a graphic display of a patient's invasive BP reading. The waveform should have a rapid, steep ascent followed by
a gradual, prolonged descent. The arterial waveform follows the QRS complex of the patient's electrocardiogram (ECG).

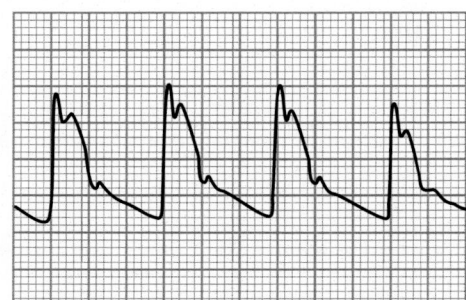

What You NEED TO KNOW

The top of the arterial waveform tracing represents the peak of systolic pressure, which depicts the contraction of the left ventricle. Next, the waveform
begins to drop; a slight increase (upstroke) is then observed in the waveform,
which is known as the dicrotic notch and depicts the closure of the aortic
valve and retrograde blood flow. Last, the waveform continues to diminish
(drop), which depicts the opening of the aortic valve and is the lowest pressure in the arterial system and is known as the end-diastolic pressure.

Answer: 5. infection and hemorrhage.

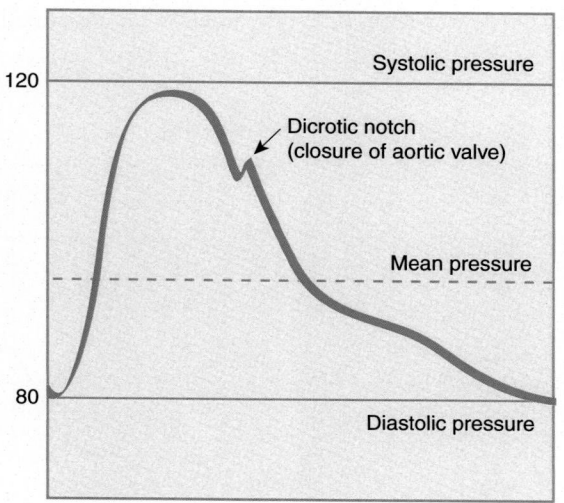

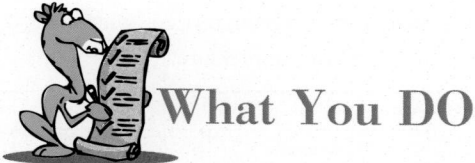

What You DO

Once the arterial line is placed and continuous monitoring is implemented, the nurse is responsible for monitoring the patient and arterial waveform and making the appropriate assessments and clinical decisions. Hemodynamic monitoring systems and equipment develop problems that could lead to erroneous readings and inappropriate treatment decisions. Common mechanical problems that occur with arterial pressure monitoring include waveform configuration changes that result in overdamping and underdamping.

Abnormal arterial waveforms and readings can result in erroneous measurements. Treatments based on erroneous measurements may result in adverse outcomes.

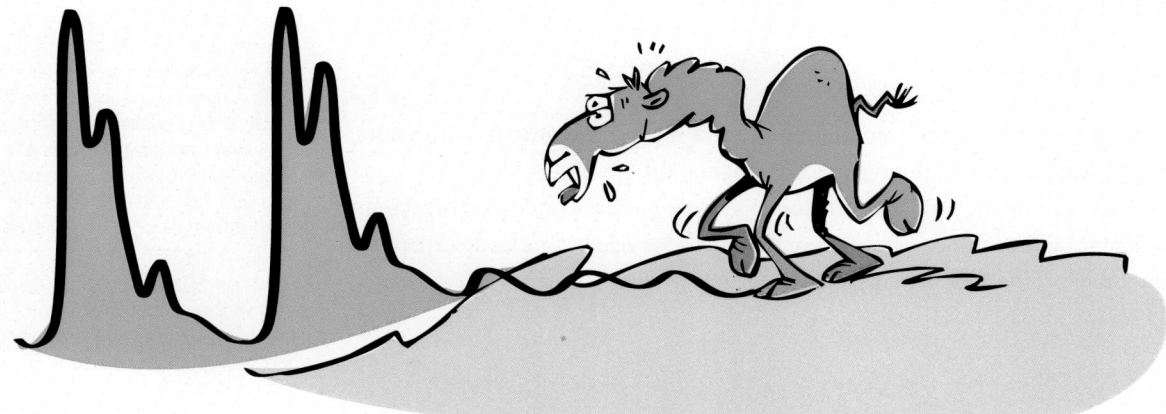

Overdamping of the waveform is best described as an unnaturally smooth waveform that loses it characteristic landmarks.

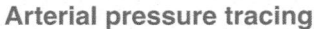

Arterial pressure tracing

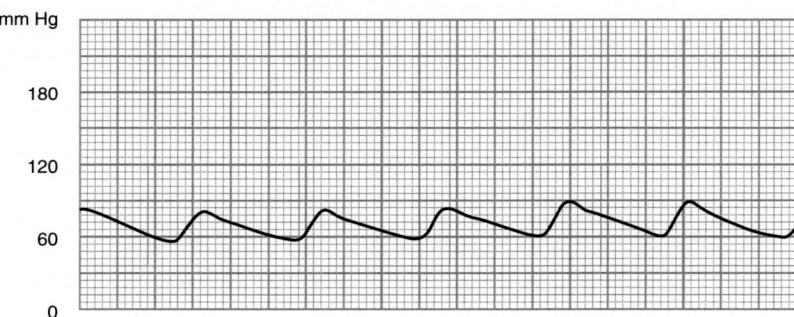

In contrast, underdamping of the waveform is characterized by an exaggeration of systolic pressure and falsely low diastolic pressure.

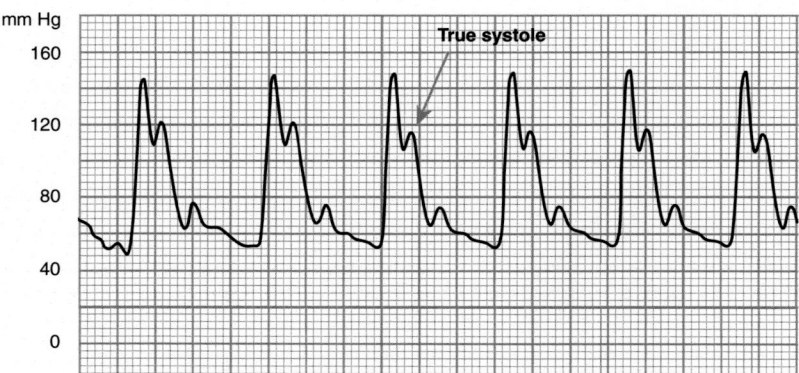

Review Chapter 3 for information on zeroing and dynamic response testing (testing for overdamping and underdamping).

Both monitoring problems are due to various patient conditions or system problems and each possess different troubleshooting actions as described in the table on the following page.

TAKE HOME POINTS

- The terms catheter fling and catheter whip actually refer to an underdamped waveform.
- Appropriately zeroing the patient's pressure monitoring system is the single most important step in obtaining accurate and meaningful data. The lines should be rezeroed every shift or when the transducer or patient position changes and when readings are in question. The catheter tip should serve as the zero reference point to the stopcock on the transducer.
- A system with appropriate dynamic response characteristics will return to the baseline pressure waveform within one to two oscillations.

Problems and Troubleshooting Arterial Monitoring

PROBLEM	CAUSE	TROUBLESHOOTING
Overdamping	• Air bubbles in the system	• Removal of excess air from flush solution bag before inserting; system completely flushed
	• Additional stopcocks	• Removal of unnecessary stopcocks
	• Catheter kink	• Examination of catheter for kinks
	• Tubing kink	• Examination of tubing for kinks
	• Blood on the transducer	• Ensurance that all connections are tightened
	• Clot in the catheter	• Maintenance of pressure on the fluid system
		• Use of correct and appropriate techniques when drawing blood from system
	• Empty flush bag	• Replacement of flush bag
	• Aortic stenosis	• Treatment of patient's condition if applicable
	• Vasodilation	
	• Low cardiac output (sepsis, hypovolemia)	
Underdamping	• Excessive tubing length (3 to 4 feet)	• Use of short, appropriate length of tubing
	• Excessive catheter movement	• Verification of optimal monitoring with performance of fast-flush square wave test
		• Immobilization and stabilization of catheter site to prevent excessive movement
	• Atherosclerosis	• Treatment of the patient's condition if applicable
	• Vasoconstriction	
	• Aortic regurgitation	
	• Hyperdynamic states (fever)	
	• Hypertension	

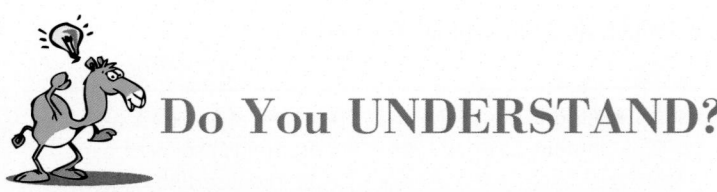

Do You UNDERSTAND?

DIRECTIONS: **Complete the following crossword puzzle.**

Down

1. Test that should be performed before puncturing or cannulating the radial artery.
2. Body fluid that can be drawn from an arterial line.
3. When doing this to medications, the arterial line provides immediate feedback on its effectiveness.
4. Insertion site that is predisposed to thrombus formation.

Down—cont'd

7. Type of waveform caused by air bubbles in the system.
8. An exaggeration of systolic pressure.
10. Arterial BP monitoring allows for this type of reading (time).

Across

5. Artery that is the most common insertion site.
6. One must make sure these are tight and not leaking to ensure that the patient does not exsanguinate.
9. Type of BP reading obtained from a cuff.
11. Arterial pressure monitoring is considered to be this type of method.
12. Notch in the waveform that represents the aortic valve being closed.
13. Patency of this artery is tested before inserting a radial catheter.
14. Another term for an underdamped waveform.

Answers: *Down:* 1. Allen; 2. blood; 3. titrating; 4. pedal; 7. overdamping; 8. underdamping; 10. continuous. *Across:* 5. radial; 6. connections; 9. indirect; 11. invasive; 12. dicrotic 13. ulnar; 14. fling.

Right Atrial and Central Venous Pressure Monitoring

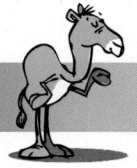

What IS Central Venous Pressure Monitoring?

Central venous pressure (CVP) is the pressure in the large thoracic veins near the right atrium. CVP directly measures the pressure in the superior vena cava (SVC) and, considering that the SVC openly communicates with the right atrium, measures right atrial pressure (RAP).

CVP normally correlates with the end-diastolic (filling) pressure of the right ventricle. As the right ventricle fills, the tricuspid valve is open, allowing open communication between the atrium and ventricle. Near the end of diastole the pressure equalizes, resulting in a reflection of the right ventricular pressure. Overall CVP reflects the relationship among the intravascular volume, venous tone, and right ventricular heart function.

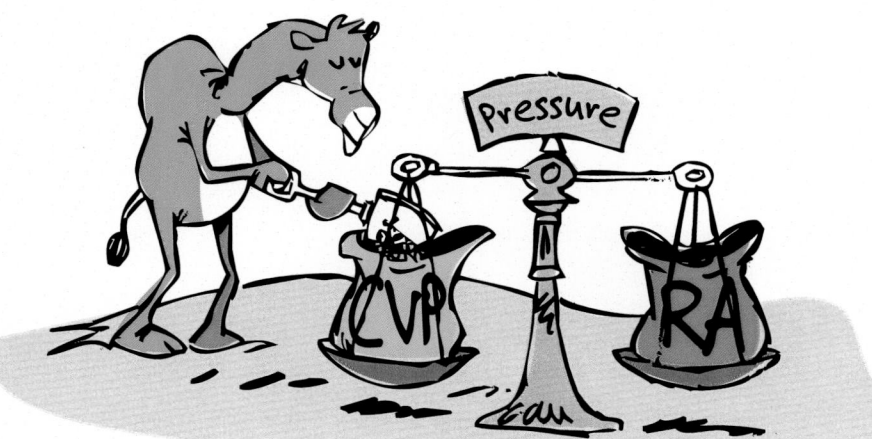

To learn more about continuous ScvO₂ monitoring, visit the Edwards Lifesciences web site at www.edwards.com.

CVP also correlates with left ventricular end–diastolic pressure in individuals without cardiovascular disease and is a means of assessing left ventricular function.

New CVP catheters have the ability to measure continuous central venous oxygen saturation ($ScvO_2$). This type of monitoring is used for the early identification of patients with global tissue oxygen deficiency (hypoxia) and early implementation of therapy.

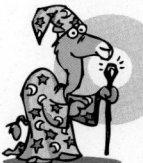

What You NEED TO KNOW

CVP monitoring is a way to measure right heart function directly and measure left heart function indirectly. Normal CVP ranges from 0 to 8 mm Hg. CVP is measured by placing a radiopaque catheter, usually via the jugular or subclavian vein, whose tip lies in the SVC near the right atrium. Serial or continuous readings provide a method for directly assessing right heart function and volume status, and indirectly assessing left heart function.

Catheters for central venous insertion are made from a variety of materials. Catheter-related complications vary with the material from which the catheter is made. For example, catheters made of polyvinyl chloride are likely to cause the most reaction in the body, possibly resulting in phlebitis or catheter-related thrombosis. Silastic catheters are more chemically inert and more flexible. However, their flexibility makes them more difficult to insert. The intended use of the catheter determines its type.

Ideally, CVP measurements should be taken with the patient supine without a pillow. However, if the patient's condition prohibits placement in the supine position, the head of the bed may be elevated up to 30 degrees. If the patient is unable to breathe when lying down (orthopneic) and cannot tolerate a position of 30 degrees or less, measure CVP in the patient's position of comfort until the orthopnea resolves.

If the patient's clinical condition prohibits placing him or her flat, document the position of the patient when the reading is obtained. Serial readings may be obtained with the patient in the same position to establish a trend. CVPs will be lower if the patient is in an upright position as a result of gravity-related changes in the intrathoracic blood volume. Variations in patient position will need to be taken into consideration when interpreting the readings.

TAKE HOME POINTS

Many brands of central venous catheters are available in prepackaged kits. Nurses should be familiar with the equipment available in their institutions.

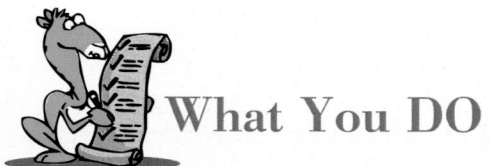

What You DO

Central venous catheters may be single lumen or multilumen. Multilumen catheters are commonly used in critical care units because when using a single-lumen catheter, fluid or drug infusions must be interrupted for CVP readings. Triple-lumen catheters have three infusion ports that terminate 2.2 cm apart at the distal end of the catheter. If a percutaneous sheath introducer with side-arm infusion port is used, a fourth lumen is available. The multiple-lumen catheters provide a mechanism for simultaneous fluid and drug administration, as well as continuous CVP monitoring. The patient's physician will select the type of catheter required by the patient's condition.

Central venous catheters are most often inserted via the jugular or subclavian vein. The femoral vein may be used, especially if the patient has coagulopathy, because the femoral site may be directly compressed if the artery is lacerated. Of the three veins, the femoral site is the least commonly used because of the increased risk of catheter-related sepsis and the need to keep the patient's leg relatively straight. The following discussion relates to the jugular and subclavian sites because these veins are most commonly used. Ideally, one nurse should be available to assist the physician and one should be available to "circulate" or monitor the patient.

Before the catheter insertion procedure, the nurse should:

- Prepare the patient and family. Explain the purpose for the central catheter and the procedure in simple nontechnical terms.
- Obtain a signed consent if required by the facility.
- Assemble the appropriate equipment (see Chapter 3).
- Place the patient supine in a Trendelenburg position of 15 to 30 degrees, unless this placement is contraindicated by the patient's condition. The Trendelenburg position promotes distension of the veins of the chest, neck, and head, making venous cannulation easier.
- Instruct cooperative patients on how to perform a Valsalva maneuver before the procedure.

Having the patient perform the Valsalva maneuver at appropriate times during the procedure and placing the patient in the Trendelenburg position reduces the risk of air embolus.

- Consider and provide, if necessary, preprocedure sedation for restless patients.

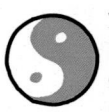
When preparing the patient and family, consider any cultural or religious beliefs that may influence the patient's understanding and attitudes about the procedure.

TAKE HOME POINTS

The Valsalva maneuver is forced exhalation against a closed glottis, similar to bearing down to have a bowel movement. The Valsalva maneuver increases intrathoracic pressure.

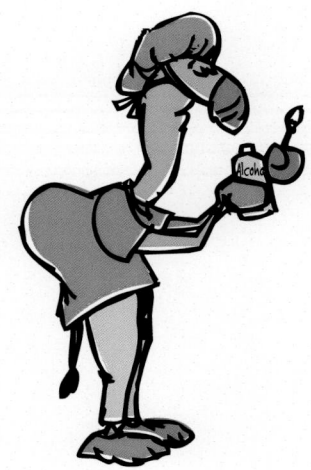

Tension pneumothorax and air embolus are two life-threatening complications of central venous catheter insertion. Both produce profound respiratory and circulatory compromise. The placement of a chest tube to remove the air from the pleural cavity is the treatment for tension pneumothorax. If the patient's condition does not allow time for the placement of a chest tube, a large-bore needle may be inserted in the second intercostal space over the rib. Immediate treatment of an air embolus includes placing the patient on their left side in the Trendelenburg position and providing 100% oxygen.

TAKE HOME POINTS

The phlebostatic axis, which is approximately at the level of the right atrium, is located at the fourth intercostal space, midway between the anterior and posterior aspects of the chest (midaxillary position).

- Discontinue feeding the patient with nasogastric tube feeding at least 10 minutes before the procedure to allow for gastric emptying, which will reduce the risk of aspiration of gastric contents during the procedure.
- Follow surgical aseptic techniques to reduce the chances of infection:
  - Operating physician and assistants must perform a full surgical scrub and don full surgical attire, gowns, gloves, caps, and masks.
  - Circulating staff and all others entering the room must wear caps and masks.
  - Cap must be placed over the patient's hair.
  - Insertion site is shaved if indicated.
  - Insertion site is cleaned with antiseptic scrub for 2 to 3 minutes.
  - Patient's head is turned in the direction opposite of the insertion site with chin pointed slightly upward.
  - Site is draped with at least a half-body drape, including covering the patient's face.

The circulating nurse is responsible for care of the patient during the procedure. The circulating nurse should:
- Obtain baseline vital signs before the start of the procedure.
- Monitor the patient closely during the procedure, including heart rate, rhythm, and blood pressure (BP).
- Immediately notify the operating physician of a change in the patient's condition.
- Obtain a chest x-ray film after the procedure to confirm catheter placement. Do not begin any intravenous (IV) fluid or flush the catheter until proper placement has been confirmed.
- Talk to the patient, and explain what is being done during the procedure. It is important to provide emotional support for the patient. Even if the patient is confused or comatose, an explanation of what is happening during the procedure is important. Reassuring words and touching the patient (e.g., holding the patient's hand) during the procedure may dramatically reduce anxiety.

To take CVP measurements, the nurse should:
- Place the patient supine and remove pillow if tolerated.
- Take the CVP reading as close to the level of the right atrium as possible. Place the zero level of the water manometer or the transducer at the phlebostatic axis.
- Obtain the reading.
- Document reading and patient position in the medical record.

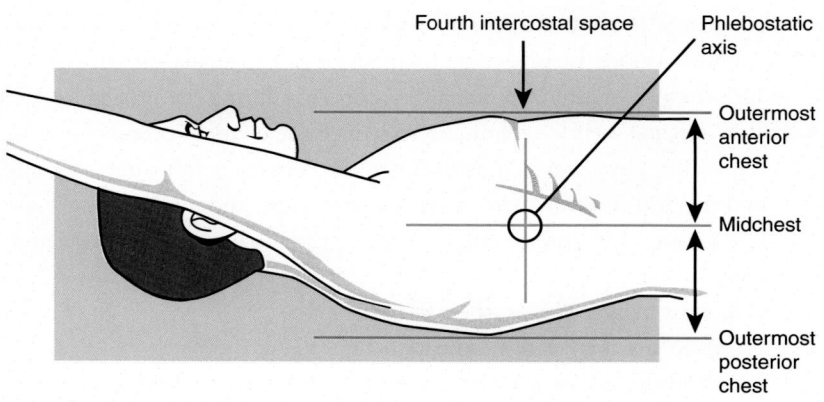

Fourth intercostal space

Phlebostatic axis

Outermost anterior chest

Midchest

Outermost posterior chest

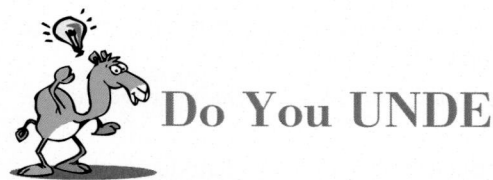

Do You UNDERSTAND?

DIRECTIONS: **Fill in the blanks to complete each of the following statements.**

1. CVP directly measures _____.

2. CVP normally correlates with the end–diastolic pressure of the

_____ _____.

3. In persons with normal hearts and lungs, CVP correlates to

_____ _____

_____–_____.

4. Normal CVP ranges from _____ to _____ mm Hg.

DIRECTIONS: **Select the best answer and place the corresponding letter in the space provided.**

_____ 5. The type of catheter used for central venous cannulation is
     a. Determined by what type is available.
     b. Selected by the nurse.
     c. Determined by the intended use.
     d. Determined by the flexibility of the catheter.

_____ 6. What is the major advantage of a multilumen catheter over a single-lumen catheter?
     a. Multilumen catheters are easier to place.
     b. Multilumen catheters allow for the simultaneous administration of fluids and continuous CVP monitoring.
     c. Multilumen catheters may be left in place for a longer time.
     d. Multilumen catheters cause fewer complications such as phlebitis.

_____ 7. Insertion of a central venous catheter is a(an)
     a. Sterile procedure.
     b. Clean procedure.
     c. Procedure that must be performed in the surgical unit.
     d. Emergency procedure.

_____ 8. The circulating nurse is responsible for
     a. Assisting the physician with the procedure.
     b. Gathering extra supplies.
     c. Maintaining the sterile field.
     d. Monitoring and comforting the patient.

_____ 9. Ideally, CVP readings should be obtained with the patient in a(an)
     a. Supine position.
     b. Elevated position.
     c. Position of comfort.
     d. Sidelying position.

_____ 10. The zero level of a water manometer or the transducer should be placed at the
     a. Midaxillary line.
     b. Level of the left ventricle.
     c. Level of the entry point of the central catheter.
     d. Phlebostatic axis.

Answers: 5. c; 6. b; 7. a; 8. d; 9. a; 10. d.

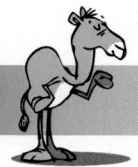

What IS Measuring CVP with a Pressure Transducer?

In current clinical practice, CVP is typically measured with the use of a pressure transducer. A pressure waveform is available for analysis, and a continuous readout is available. All hemodynamic monitoring equipment consists of a transducer, an amplifier, a display module, and a fluid-filled catheter. The transducer senses a physiologic event and transforms it into electrical signals. The amplifier amplifies and filters out interference and transmits the signal to the display module. The catheter and flush system maintain the patency of the catheter. (See Chapter 3 for more information on monitoring equipment.)

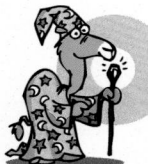

What You NEED TO KNOW

When measuring CVP with a pressure transducer, a continuous RAP tracing will be observed on the monitor. Three upward deflections typically correspond to phases of the cardiac cycle. The *a* wave is produced with atrial contraction. Enlarged *a* waves may indicate right ventricular failure of any cause. In atrial fibrillation or flutter, *a* waves may be absent. The *c* wave is produced when the tricuspid valve closes. The bulging of the tricuspid valve into the right atrium as the right ventricle contracts produces the *v* wave. Large *v* waves may indicate tricuspid regurgitation. The downward deflections, the *x* and *y* waves, depict atrial diastole and emptying, respectively.

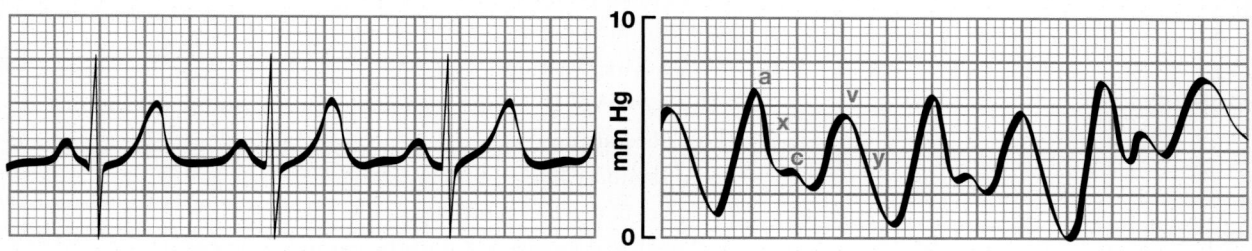

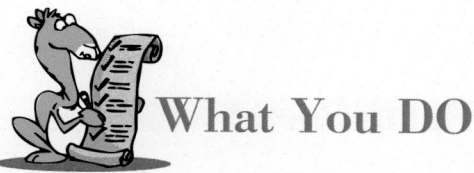

What You DO

To obtain CVP readings with a transducer setup, the nurse should:

- Wash hands.
- Validate the RAP waveform on the monitor to ensure proper catheter location.
- Fast flush the catheter for 2 seconds to ensure catheter patency.
- Ensure that the transducer is at the level of the phlebostatic axis.
- Print out at least three respiratory cycles of the waveform.
- Identify the end-expiratory phase of each respiratory cycle, and find two cycles where the end-expiratory phase is the same point, which is the CVP (RAP).
- Wash hands. To promote consistency in interpretation, record in the medical record the CVP (RAP) in mm Hg, the patient's body position, and the point on the printout where the reading was taken. Place the strip in the medical record.

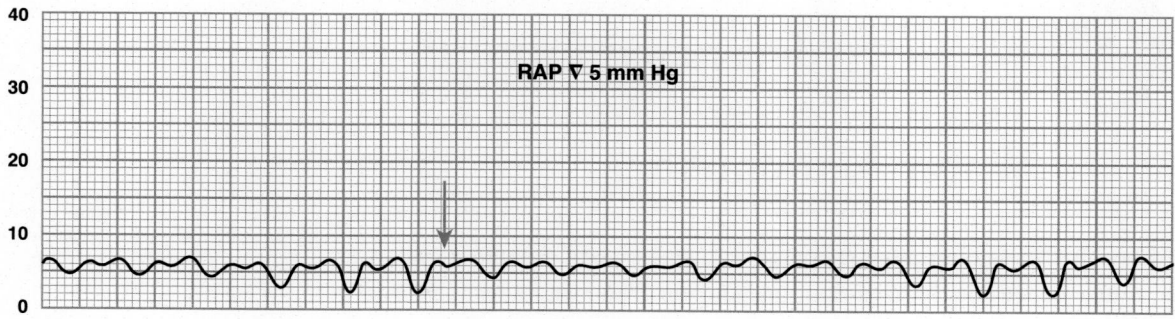

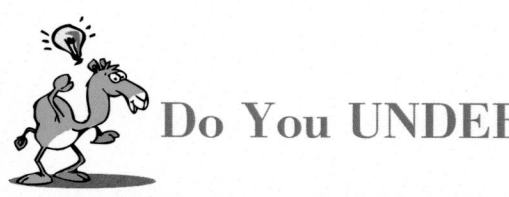

Do You UNDERSTAND?

DIRECTIONS: **Match each statement in Column A with the appropriate answer in Column B.**

Column A

_____ 1. CVP measured with a pressure transducer gives a _____.

_____ 2. The RAP is measured _____.

_____ 3. The *a* wave corresponds to _____.

_____ 4. The *c* wave is produced by _____.

_____ 5. The *v* wave is produced by _____.

Column B

a. Right ventricular contraction

b. Continuous printout

c. Tricuspid valve closure

d. Right atrial contraction

e. At the end of expiration

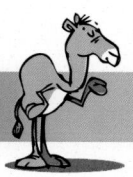

What IS Measuring Central Venous Pressure with a Water Manometer?

Although CVP is most often measured with the use of a pressure transducer, it may be measured with a water manometer. The major advantage to a water manometer is its simplicity and quick set-up time. The water manometer is attached in line with the IV fluid administration set and comes with a preattached stopcock. When the stopcock is "off" to the manometer, the IV fluid may flow freely to the patient. When measuring CVP the nurse may attach the water manometer to the IV pole, level it with the phlebostatic axis using a carpenter's level, and measure readings with the manometer on the pole. The nurse may also remove the manometer from the pole and hold it at the phlebostatic axis for each reading.

Answers: 1. b; 2. e; 3. d; 4. c; 5. a.

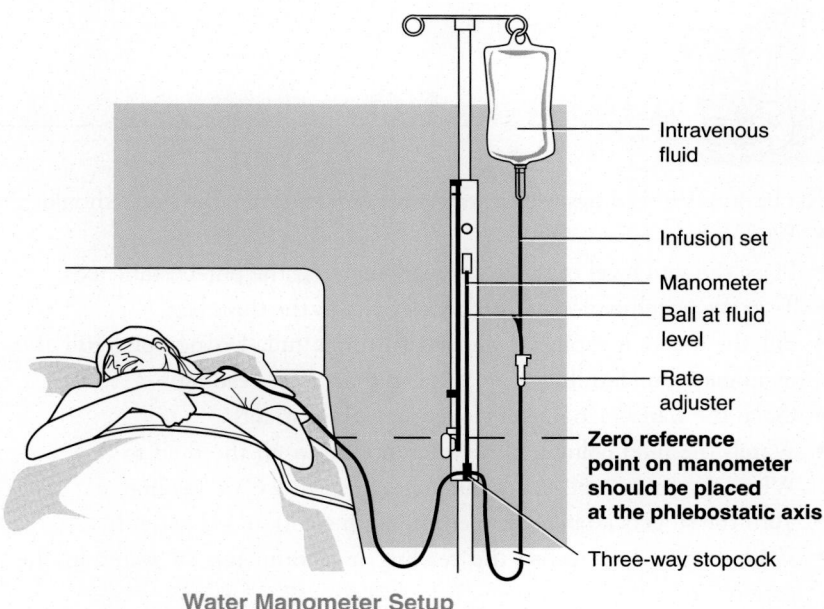

Water Manometer Setup

- Intravenous fluid
- Infusion set
- Manometer
- Ball at fluid level
- Rate adjuster
- **Zero reference point on manometer should be placed at the phlebostatic axis**
- Three-way stopcock

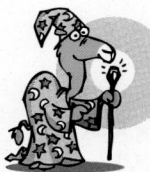

What You NEED TO KNOW

Continuous reading is not possible with a water manometer. Serial readings must be obtained on a regular basis and the trend is documented to provide information for making treatment decisions.

Water manometers function by filling the chamber with IV fluid, opening the chamber to the patient, and allowing the fluid level to equalize with the pressure in the right atrium. Once the manometer is open to the patient, the level will fall rapidly. The column of water should stop falling and fluctuate when the pressure equalizes with the RAP, which is the CVP reading. The water column may fluctuate with respirations, making exact reading difficult. Readings are noted in centimeters of water.

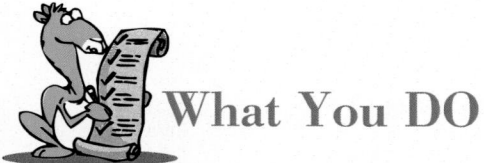

What You DO

To obtain CVP readings with a water manometer setup, the nurse should:
- Wash hands.
- Place the zero level of the water manometer at the phlebostatic axis.
- Turn the water manometer stopcock open to the flush bag.
- Fill the water manometer about two-thirds full. Do not underfill the manometer; underfilling may cause an inaccurate reading.
- Open the water manometer stopcock to the patient.
- Watch the fluid column closely. Do not allow all the fluid to flow out. When the column begins to fluctuate, this is the CVP reading.
- Turn the stopcock open between the flush solution and patient.
- Wash hands, and record the reading in centimeters of water in the patient's record.

- **Do not allow fluid to overflow from the top of the manometer. This overflow will result in contamination.**
- **Do not allow all the fluid to run out of the manometer. Doing so could cause an air embolus.**

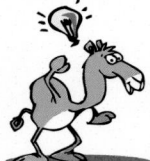

Do You UNDERSTAND?

DIRECTIONS: **Identify the following statements as** *true* **(T) or** *false* **(F).**

_____ 1. Water manometers are commonly used to measure CVP.

_____ 2. Continuous CVP reading is possible with a water manometer.

_____ 3. To prevent air embolus, it is important that the nurse does not allow all the fluid to flow out of the water manometer.

_____ 4. The CVP reading should be obtained when the fluid column fluctuates.

Answers: 1. F; 2. F; 3. T; 4. T.

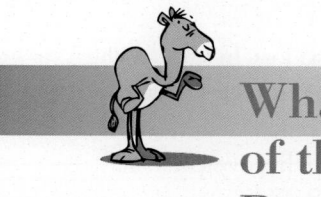

What IS the Meaning of the Central Venous Pressure Reading?

CVP is the pressure in the large thoracic vessels of the chest and reflects the pressure in the right side of the heart. CVP is a reflection of right ventricular end–diastolic pressure or preload. Alterations in preload affect cardiac output. Abnormal CVP may indicate altered right heart function and volume status. It is important to remember that an isolated CVP reading is not as valuable as a series of readings. The trend of the CVP will communicate more about the patient's condition.

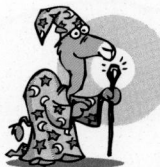

What You NEED TO KNOW

CVP measurements are most often used to assess and manage intravascular volume status. Alterations in CVP most directly reflect right-sided heart function. Increased CVP may indicate any of the following:

- Intravascular volume overload
- Cardiac tamponade or pericardial effusion
- Right-sided valve disease
- Right ventricular failure secondary to left heart failure such as myocardial infarction, mitral or aortic stenosis, or cardiomyopathy
- Right ventricular failure secondary to increased pulmonary vascular resistance
- Right ventricular failure as a result of right ventricular infarction or cardiomyopathy

A significantly increased CVP often indicates volume overload. Volume overload may result from overaggressive IV fluid administration. Other reasons that may cause an elevated CVP relate to conditions that overload the right ventricle (e.g., pulmonary hypertension or right ventricular failure), causing the right ventricle to be unable to eject properly. Decreased CVP may indicate:

- Hypovolemia
- Alteration in venous tone

Hypovolemia may be the result of dehydration or blood loss. In states such as septic shock, extreme vasodilatation occurs, resulting in relative hypovolemia. In this state the poor venous tone causes poor venous return to the heart, mimicking a hypovolemic state. Other signs of hypovolemia may include elevated heart rate, decreased BP, and decreased urine output.

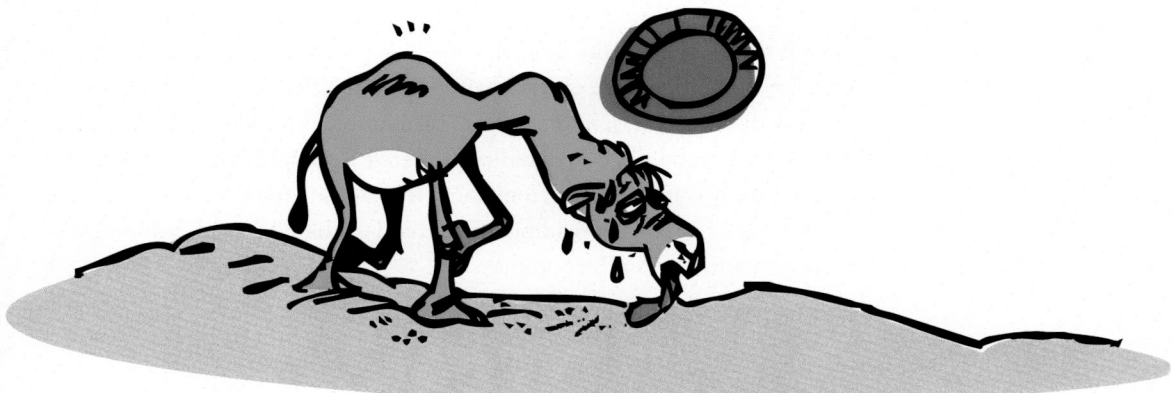

A normal CVP does not necessarily mean that the patient has a normal volume status. Compensatory mechanisms can keep cardiac output at normal levels at least temporarily. A patient taking vasoactive drugs may have a normal or elevated CVP even in a hypovolemic state.

Mechanical ventilation may falsely elevate CVP readings. Positive pressure ventilator breaths increase atrial pressure, impede venous return, and therefore decrease cardiac output. The use of positive end–expiratory pressure (PEEP) further increases intrathoracic pressure, often causing unpredictable CVP readings. However, it is not clinically sound to remove patients from mechanical ventilation to obtain CVP readings, especially patients who are on PEEP.

TAKE HOME POINTS

CVP readings of mechanically ventilated patients that do not correlate with the patient's clinical picture might be false.

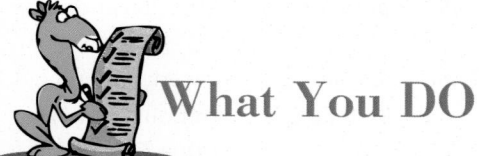 **What You DO**

If hypovolemia is suspected, the clinical response to fluid challenges are more meaningful than isolated CVP readings. A rapid infusion of 300 to 500 ml fluid in a normovolemic healthy adult will increase the CVP by 2 to 4 mm Hg. The reading will return to baseline in 10 to 15 minutes. A CVP that does not return to baseline in 10 minutes indicates increased intravascular volume, a noncompliant right ventricle, or both. Hypovolemia is possible if the CVP fails to increase or return to baseline in 5 minutes.

Common Complications of CVP Monitoring and Appropriate Nursing Responses

COMPLICATIONS	BACKGROUND INFORMATION	NURSING RESPONSIBILITIES
Hemorrhage	• Overt hemorrhage may occur from the insertion site. • Occult bleeding may occur into a body cavity or cause a deep-tissue hematoma.	• Check for visible signs of bleeding such as bruising or swelling. Apply pressure as appropriate. • Monitor the patient for signs of occult bleeding such as hypovolemia, restlessness, pallor, cool distal extremities, and tachycardia.
Pneumothorax	• Increased incidence may occur when the subclavian vein is cannulated. • Increased incidence may occur when patient is on mechanical ventilation, especially PEEP. • Occurs on insertion. • Overall incidence is 1% to 2%.	• Monitor patient for dyspnea, cough, and sharp chest pain. • Confirm with chest x-ray film. • Assist with chest tube placement.
Vascular erosions	• Occurs 1 to 7 days after insertion. • Caused by vessel wall irritation by stiff catheter or infusion of caustic or hypertonic solutions. • May cause accumulation of IV solution or blood in the pleural space or mediastinum.	• Watch for new pleural effusion or widening of mediastinum on chest x-ray. • Monitor patient for sudden onset of dyspnea, tachypnea, or tachycardia.
Dysrhythmia	• Caused by irritation of the right atrium or ventricle as a result of catheter migration. • Ventricular ectopy may occur when patient is turned; may stop when patient is returned to original position.	• Easily documented in chest x-ray. • Physician must reposition catheter.
Infection	• May occur as a result of contamination during insertion, inward catheter migration, colonization from another infected area, contaminated tubing, or IV fluids. • May be local or systemic.	• Monitor patient for fever or hypothermia, chills, localized redness, swelling, heat, purulent drainage or pain at or above the insertion site, and unexplained escalation of white blood count.

Complications of CVP monitoring are essentially the same as those associated with any central venous access. The most common complications and the appropriate nursing responses are listed in the above table.

Common Complications of CVP Monitoring and Appropriate Nursing Responses—cont'd

COMPLICATIONS	BACKGROUND INFORMATION	NURSING RESPONSIBILITIES
Fluid overload or hypothermia	• Caused by unregulated IV fluid bolus. • Relatively small amounts of fluid that are accidentally infused may be hazardous to the critically ill patient.	• Monitor patient for tachypnea, dyspnea, hypertension, and pulmonary edema. • Forced diuresis for fluid overload may be needed. • To prevent hypothermia, administer warm IV fluids if large amounts of fluids are to be infused.
Thromboembolic complications	• Catheter lumen may become occluded by blood clot. • A clot may surround one segment or all of the catheter. • Migration of a clot may result in pulmonary embolus.	• Do not force flush a central venous catheter to prevent dislodging a clot. • If one port of a multilumen catheter is not in use, intermittent flushes may help prevent thrombus formation. • Treatment requires anticoagulant therapy.
Air embolus	• Air may enter the vascular system during catheter insertion, removal, or any time during which the tubing is being disconnected. • Cardiovascular collapse and death may result.	• Teach alert patients Valsalva maneuver. • Make sure all tubing and catheter connections are secure. • Monitor patient for sudden cyanosis, tachypnea, tachycardia, and hypotension. • Immediate therapy is to place patient on left side and administer 100% oxygen.

PEEP, Positive end–expiratory pressure.

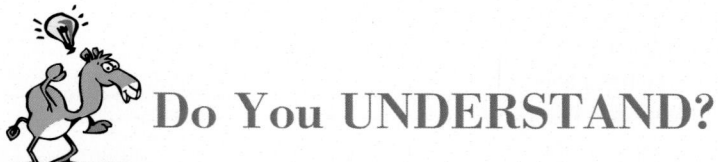

Do You UNDERSTAND?

DIRECTIONS: **Fill in the blanks to complete the following statements.**

1. Decisions about treatment of the patient should be based on the

_____.

2. Low CVP readings may be an indication of _____.

3. Clinical response to a _____ _____

is more meaningful than an isolated CVP reading.

4. Mechanical ventilation may _____ CVP readings.

DIRECTIONS: **Select the appropriate answer or answers for each question, and place the corresponding letter or letters in the space provided.**

_____ 5. Infection may be caused by
   a. Contamination during insertion.
   b. Inward catheter migration.
   c. Contaminated tubing.
   d. All of the above.
_____ 6. Air embolus may be a life-threatening complication.
   a. True
   b. False
_____ 7. Pneumothorax usually occurs
   a. 1 to 7 days after insertion.
   b. Immediately after insertion when the subclavian site is used.
   c. After long-term central venous therapy.
   d. Immediately after insertion when the jugular site is used.

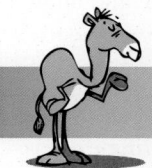

What IS Central Venous Catheter Removal?

Central venous catheters may be removed for a number of reasons. The most positive reason for catheter removal is that the patient's condition has improved and the central venous catheter is no longer needed. Catheters may also be removed if they become damaged or the patient develops an infection. The infection may be systemic or localized at the catheter insertion site. If the catheter must be removed because of damage or infection and the patient's condition continues to warrant the need for the catheter, the physician may choose to place a new catheter in a different location.

Answers: 3. fluid challenge; 4. alter; 5. d; 6. a; 7. b.

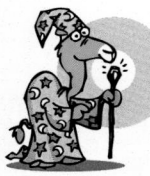

What You NEED TO KNOW

When removing a central venous catheter, correct technique is critical. Air embolus is a complication of central venous catheter removal. It is important to remove the catheter while the patient is performing a Valsalva maneuver when there is positive intrathoracic pressure. During removal, resistance should be minimal. If significant resistance is met during removal, stop the procedure and assess with an x-ray film. The catheter may be knotted or kinked.

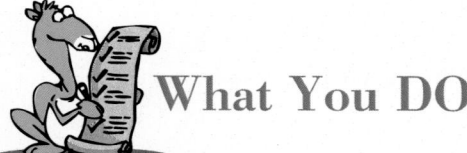

What You DO

To remove a central venous catheter, the nurse should:
- Explain the procedure to the patient.
- Wash hands.
- Place patient in a supine or Trendelenburg position.
- Close all catheter ports.
- Remove the dressing and clean the site with povidone-iodine and allow to dry.
- Cut the sutures.
- Have the cooperative patient perform the Valsalva maneuver during the 3 to 5 seconds of catheter removal. Remove the catheter during expiration if the patient is not cooperative. Remove the catheter during midinspiration if the patient is mechanically ventilated.
- Apply pressure to the insertion site for 5 to 15 minutes to stop bleeding once the catheter is removed.
- Apply an occlusive dressing after hemostasis is obtained.
- Ensure that the patient remains in bed for 15 to 30 minutes after the procedure.

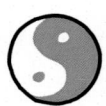
While preparing the patient, consider any cultural or religious beliefs that may influence the patient's understanding and attitudes about the procedure.

If significant resistance is met during catheter removal, stop the procedure and assess with an x-ray film. The catheter may be knotted or kinked.

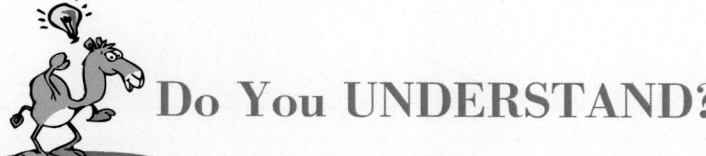

Do You UNDERSTAND?

DIRECTIONS: **Select the best answer for each statement, and place the corresponding letter in the space provided.**

_____ 1. One complication of central venous catheter removal is
     a. Air embolus.
     b. Infection.
     c. Hemorrhage.
     d. Fat embolus.

_____ 2. If significant resistance is met when removing a central venous catheter,
     a. Pull harder.
     b. Apply a more steady pressure.
     c. Stop and obtain a chest x-ray.
     d. Advance the catheter.

Answers: 1. a; 2. c

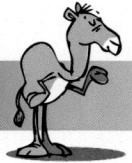

CHAPTER 6
Pulmonary Artery Pressure Monitoring

What IS Pulmonary Artery Pressure Monitoring?

Pulmonary artery (PA) pressure monitoring is the monitoring of the pressures within the PA leading to the lungs. Just as an arterial line provides a direct reflection of systemic blood pressure, a PA line provides a reflection of pulmonary blood pressure. In addition to direct measurement of lung pressures, the catheter allows indirect measurements of left heart pressures and provides information necessary for calculating cardiac output (CO) and blood vessel status. PA pressure monitoring can assess all three components of stroke volume—preload, afterload, and contractility.

The PA catheter is a long, hollow, flexible catheter (usually yellow) with multiple pigtails and corresponding lumens or tunnels. The most commonly used type is a quad-lumen 7 Fr thermodilution catheter. (See Color Plate 4.)

The PA catheter is marked with encircling black lines to allow estimation of catheter tip location. Each thin black line equals 10 cm; the heavy black line is 50 cm. The catheter has multiple lumens, each with unique functions.

Distal Port

The distal port:
- Terminates in the PA.
- Must be connected before floating the catheter into the PA.
- Connects to a stopcock and to pressure transducer tubing.

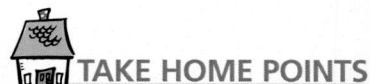

TAKE HOME POINTS

Before the nurse can understand PA monitoring, he or she must first understand cardiac anatomy and hemodynamic theory. (Review Chapters 1 and 2 if these points remain unclear.)

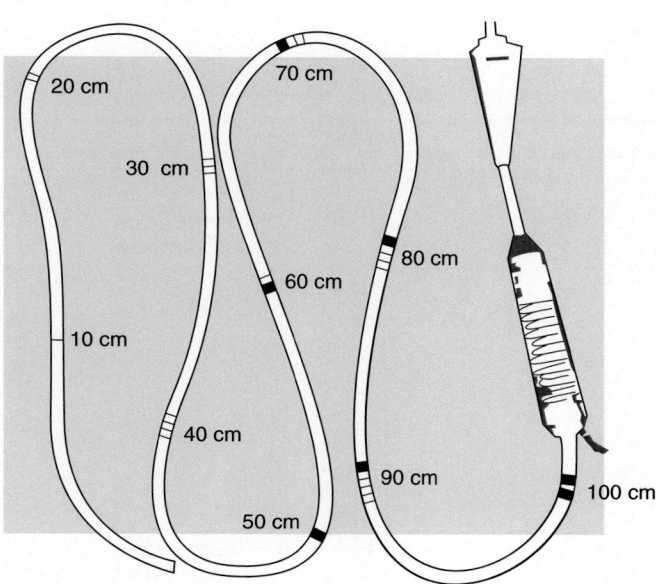

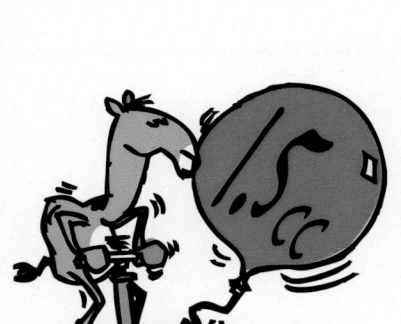

Fluids and medica-
tions are NOT infused
or directly pushed
through the intravenous (IV)
distal port because the tip
terminates in the PA, leading
directly into the lungs.

- Is used for monitoring PA pressures.
- Provides a port for drawing mixed venous blood gases.

Balloon Inflation Port

The balloon inflation port:

- Is equipped with a valve that enables a tiny balloon at the tip of the catheter to be inflated with a special syringe. The syringe will not allow injection of greater than $1^1/_2$ ml air.
- Has a locking device for safety.
- Is inflated during insertion of the catheter to allow the catheter tip to flow through the various cardiac structures without causing damage to the cardiac tissue.
- Is used to measure pulmonary artery occlusion pressures (PAOP) (also referred to as pulmonary capillary wedge pressure [PCWP]) by periodically inflating to allow it to "wedge" into a smaller branch of an arteriole. Balloon inflation allows the catheter to measure pressure in the pulmonary capillary bed, which is equal to the pressure in both the left atrium and left ventricle during diastole. (See Chapter 7 for a more thorough discussion of PAOP.)

Close-up of catheter tip

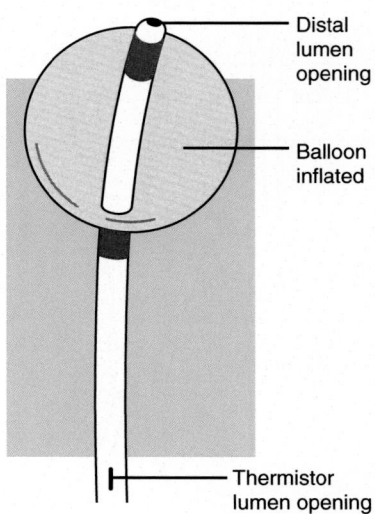

Distal
lumen
opening

Balloon
inflated

Thermistor
lumen opening

Use only the syringe provided with the PA catheter to inflate the balloon. Overinflation with a larger syringe can cause the balloon to rupture.

Proximal Injectate Port

The proximal injectate port:
- Is blue in color.
- Provides a port for injecting fluid for measuring CO.
- Measures the central venous pressure (CVP) by being connected to a pressure transducer and tubing.
- May infuse IV fluids if continuous measurement of CVP is not necessary.
- Can infuse vasoactive or inotropic agents if not being used for measuring CO.

Proximal Infusion Port

The proximal infusion port:
- Is white in color; is also the venous infusion port (VIP).
- Provides an extra port whose lumen also opens in the right atrium (RA).
- Provides a central line to infuse all types of fluid or medication or both without interrupting CO measurement.
- Is not attached to a pressure transducer.
- May be a newer version that has a second VIP located in the right ventricle (RV).

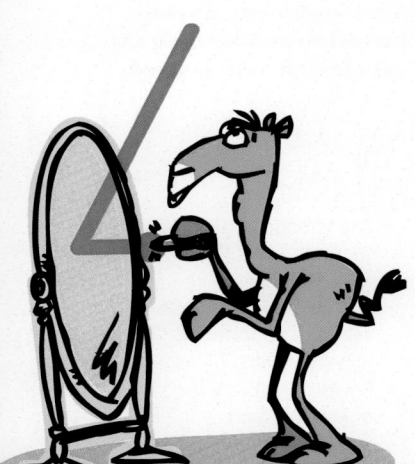

Cardiac Output Port

The cardiac output port:

- Is a white, square port containing several pins for inserting into the CO cable.
- Locks into the monitor cable connected to the bedside monitor.
- Provides temperature-sensitive wires that extend through the catheter and terminate in a thermistor sensor, which is close to the distal tip.
- Is used for *thermodilution* measurement of CO.

Other Ports (Optional)

- Pace-Port for a ventricular or atrial pacemaker. This lumen terminates in the RV or RA and is to be used for pacing if needed.
- Continuous venous oxygen saturation (SvO_2) monitoring via fiberoptics. This type of port transmits a tiny beam of light through the catheter and into the PA circulation. Oxygen levels determine how much blood reflects the light; the amount of blood is registered back to the monitor as a digital readout.

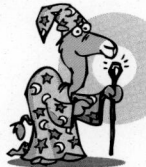

What You NEED TO KNOW

The delivery of oxygen to the tissues depends largely on the delicate interplay among blood volume, vessel tone, and the heart's pumping action. Hemodynamic monitoring is a way of assessing each part of this process. The blood volume (preload), the vessel tone (afterload), and the heart's pumping action (contractility) can be measured by inserting a catheter into the PA.

The PA catheter is inserted via the central venous system into the heart. On insertion, the tip of the catheter is passed through the RA to the RV through the pulmonary valve into the PA. The distal tip of the catheter, once inserted, rests in the PA. It continually measures pressures from the right side of the heart and lungs (PA systolic and diastolic), which are helpful in detecting certain *right*-sided pulmonary or cardiac conditions. However, a PA catheter is usually inserted to indirectly measure *left*-sided pressures. This measuring function is accomplished by inflating the balloon on the catheter tip. Balloon inflation allows the tip to float out to a more distal branch of a pulmonary arteriole until the size of the balloon equals the size of the blood vessel. This is called the *wedge pressure* (PCWP or PAOP).

A PA catheter can be inserted at the bedside without using fluoroscopy. It is usually inserted into a large diameter central vein, such as the internal jugular or subclavian vein. The patient's left side may be preferred for insertion because the venous anatomy on the left allows balloon tip flotation more easily into the RV. Typically, the PA catheter is placed into a percutaneously inserted introducer sheath with a sterile sleeve. The sleeve maintains the sterility of the catheter if manipulation is necessary after insertion.

Catheter insertion should be reserved for patients who may gain the maximum benefit. The catheter should only be inserted when there are skilled bedside clinicians trained to monitor and treat the data obtained.

Indications

PA pressure monitoring is indicated in the following situations:
- To assist in making a differential diagnosis, enabling the parameters of CO to be appropriately treated.
- To guide the clinical management of several heart and lung disorders.
- To monitor hemodynamic pressures during volume resuscitation and inotropic, vasopressor, or vasodilator drug infusion therapy.
- To assess complications of myocardial infarction and heart failure.
- To monitor hemodynamic pressures in complicated surgical procedures.

Contraindications

Although there are no absolute contraindications to the insertion of a PA catheter, relative contraindications exist for patients:
- With severe coagulopathies.
- Receiving thrombolytic therapy.
- With prosthetic right heart valves.
- With endocardial pacemakers.
- With severe pulmonary hypertension.
- With severe vascular disease.

Waveform Analysis

To understand the pressures associated with the insertion of a PA catheter, familiarity with the waveforms of each heart chamber and the vessel that the catheter must pass through is necessary. These waveforms include those of the RA, RV, PA, and PAOP. The configuration during PA catheter insertion should look like the waveform on the following page.

Because of the proximity to the apex of the lungs, the risk of the catheter puncturing the lung and causing a pneumothorax during insertion exists when the subclavian vein is used.

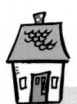

TAKE HOME POINTS
- The femoral vein may also be used to insert a PA catheter.
- No risk of pneumothorax exists at this site; but because the femoral vein is more tortuous, fluoroscopy may be needed for visualization.
- Review Chapter 5 for a more thorough discussion of the RA and CVP waveforms.
- Review Chapter 7 for a more thorough discussion of RV, PA, and PAOP waveforms.

TAKE HOME POINTS

The PA catheter is sometimes called a *Swan-Ganz* catheter or a *Swan* because it was the prototype of all PA catheters. Dr. Swan and Dr. Ganz developed the PA catheter in the 1970s.

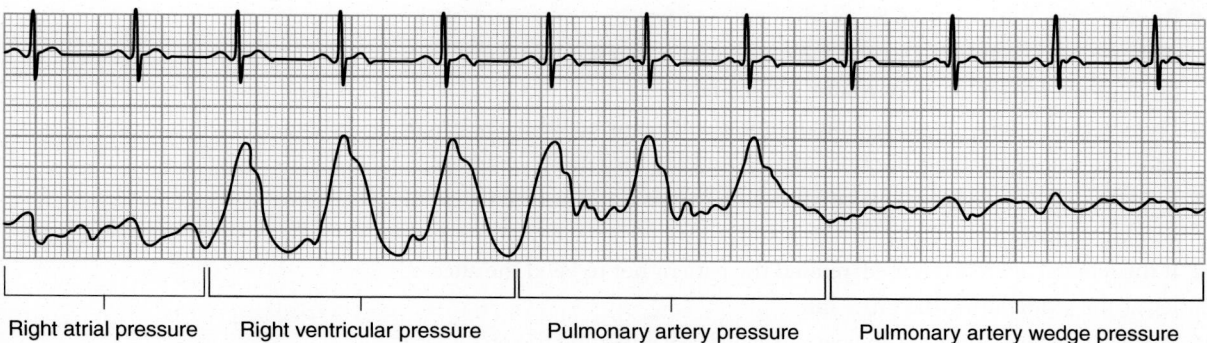

| Right atrial pressure | Right ventricular pressure | Pulmonary artery pressure | Pulmonary artery wedge pressure |

Different blood vessels and chambers within the heart and lungs generate different pressures. Waveforms are electronic depictions of these pressures. The in-line transducer on the hemodynamic setup converts the mechanical signals of the pressures within the body into electronic signals observed on the monitor as waveforms.

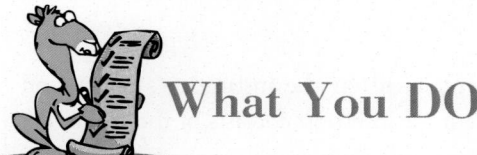

What You DO

The physician will actually insert the catheter. The nurse is responsible for preparing the patient, which includes education and IV sedation, preparing and setting up the hemodynamic monitoring equipment, assisting the physician, and monitoring the patient during the procedure.

Preparing the Patient

Before inserting the catheter, the nurse should:
- Take "time out" to verify that the correct procedure is being performed on the right patient.
- Confirm that the patient has no drug allergies.
- Confirm that the physician has explained the risks of the procedure to the patient.
- Ensure that the patient has given informed consent.
- Explain the procedure to the patient.
- Prepare the patient for the sterile nature of the procedure—the presence of the gowns, masks, and drapes, as well as the length of the procedure.
- Reassure the patient that IV sedation may be administered before the procedure to reduce anxiety.

When preparing the patient, consider any cultural or religious beliefs that may influence the patient's understanding and attitudes about the procedure.

- Reassure the patient that he or she will not feel any sensation of the catheter being advanced or the balloon being inflated. Only the needle prick of the initial local anesthetic will be felt.
- Prepare the patient for the interaction that will occur between the physician and nurses as the balloon is inflated and the monitor is observed.
- Explain that the catheter will be sutured to the skin and a sterile dressing will be applied.
- If the femoral approach is used, remind the patient not to bend the affected leg at the groin during the procedure.
- Answer any questions that the patient may have regarding the procedure.
- Lastly, include the patient's family and significant others in the education process. Take the time to give a simple explanation of the procedure and of what to expect when visiting afterward.
- Obtain the patient's baseline vital signs and oxygen saturation.

Preparing and Setting Up the Hemodynamic Monitoring Equipment

The nurse should:

- Gather the necessary equipment based on the institution's policy and procedure. In general, equipment for insertion consists of the sterile PA catheter itself, an introducer kit, sterile flush and syringes, sterile gowns, masks, drapes, gloves, and a pressure line setup (normal saline [NS] heparin flush solution, pressure tubing with three-way stopcocks, and pressure bag). (Refer to Chapter 3 for a review of equipment setup.)
- Assemble the appropriate cardules, cables, transducers, and other equipment.
- Flush the pressure tubing and transducers. (Refer to Chapter 3.)
- Calibrate and zero the transducer. (Refer to Chapter 3.)
- Ensure that the distal port is connected to the pressure tubing and transducer.
- Ensure that the side port of the transducer is level with the patient's RA.
- Discontinue tube feedings, and connect indwelling nasogastric (NG) tube to suction during the procedure.
- Have an IV port readily accessible for administering emergency IV medications.

Assisting the Physician with the Insertion Procedure

The physician will determine the site of insertion. The nurse should:

- Have the patient lie flat in bed if the femoral site is being used for insertion.

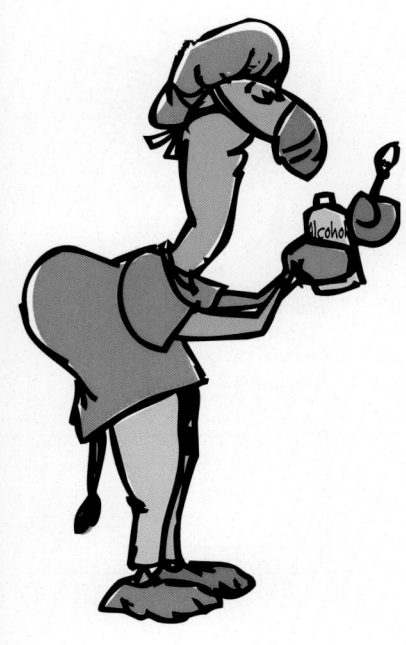

- Place the patient in the Trendelenburg position to engorge neck vessels and increase CVP if the subclavian or internal jugular site is selected for insertion. A rolled towel may need to be placed between the patient's shoulder blades to help separate the apex of the lung from the subclavian vein. This will enhance visualization of the vasculature and will decrease the risk of inadvertent pneumothorax or venous air embolism.
- Administer IV sedation to the patient at this time.
- Put on a sterile gown, mask, and gloves to assist the physician.
- The physician will drape and prepare the patient, and prepare the sterile field.
- The physician will open the PA catheter package. The physician will test the balloon by inflating it with $1^1/2$ ml air (or the full amount recommended by manufacturer). Submerging the balloon in a bowl of sterile saline may also be performed to test for leaks. The physician will then flush all lumens of the catheter with NS and heparin solution. (The nurse may be asked to assist.)
- The physician will infiltrate the site with local anesthetic.
- The physician will insert the catheter first into the sterile sleeve and then into the introducer. The physician will usually use a modified Seldinger technique to insert a large introducer catheter. This procedure involves the following steps:
  1. An initial prick is made with a locator needle.
  2. A floppy guide wire is threaded through the needle.
  3. The needle is removed.
  4. The opening is enlarged with the prick of a scalpel blade.
  5. A sheath introducer catheter is inserted over the wire.
  6. The wire is removed, leaving in only the introducer sheath.
  7. The PA catheter is inserted through the introducer sheath.

As the catheter is advanced into the RA, the nurse may be asked to inflate the balloon with the syringe. Inflating the balloon during insertion allows blood flow through the heart to direct or pull the catheter up into the PA.

Pressure at the tip of the catheter is continuously monitored as the catheter is advanced through the right heart and into the PA. As the balloon floats through each chamber, placement is confirmed by the appearance of a characteristic change in the waveform.

⚠ • **DURING insertion, always use the full amount of air prescribed (usually $1^1/2$ ml) to inflate the balloon, which prevents the hard tip from damaging blood vessels.**
- **AFTER insertion and during wedging, the balloon will be in a smaller space and therefore should be inflated with just enough air to elicit a wedge waveform (not always $1^1/2$ ml).**

Right atrial pressure
Normal range
Mean: 0-8 mm Hg
Average: 4 mm Hg

Right ventricular pressure
Normal range
Systolic: 15-30 mm Hg
Diastolic: 0-8 mm Hg
Average: 22/4 mm Hg

Pulmonary artery pressure
Normal range
Systolic: 15-30 mm Hg
Diastolic: 6-12 mm Hg
Average: 22/9 mm Hg

Pulmonary artery wedge
 pressure
Normal range
Mean: 4-12 mm Hg

During catheter insertion, some atrial irritability (premature atrial con-tractions [PACs]) may be observed when the catheter floats through the RA, and some ventricular irritability (premature ventricular contractions [PVCs] or ventricular tachycardia) may occur when the catheter floats through the RV. Both PACs and PVCs are due to mechanical irritation and should resolve spontaneously. Pressures for each chamber are recorded as the balloon passes through the RA, tricuspid valve, RV, pulmonic valve, and eventually into the PA.

During insertion—as the balloon floats from the RV to the PA—the waveform's systolic peak does not change because the RV systolic and PA systolic pressures are the same. They are the same because the pulmonic valve is open during systole. However, when the pulmonic valve closes and diastole begins, there is a slight increase in pressure. This increase is depict-ed on the waveform as the dicrotic notch. During diastole when the pul-monic valve is closed, the PA diastolic pressure is determined by resistance of the pulmonary vessels; it will be higher than the RV diastolic pressure.

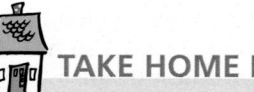

TAKE HOME POINTS

When the catheter has passed through the pulmonic valve, the characteristic dicrotic notch is observed on the waveform and the PA diastolic pressure becomes higher than the RV diastolic pressure.

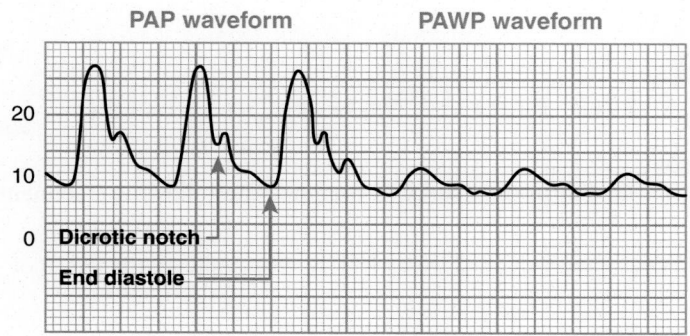

PAP waveform   PAWP waveform

20

10

0   **Dicrotic notch**
    End diastole

⚠️ **Do not leave the balloon inflated for longer than 15 seconds. A pulmonary infarct could occur!**

The balloon will continue to float until it becomes wedged. A characteristic wedge (PAOP) waveform will appear. The wedge waveform should approximate the level of the pulmonary artery diastolic (PAD) pressure. Once in the PAOP position, this number is recorded and the balloon deflated within 15 seconds, which will prevent prolonged ischemia of the pulmonary arteriole distal to the balloon.

Be prepared to print a recording of pressures measured during insertion. This will be the only opportunity to measure the RV pressure, which will only be present for a few seconds as the catheter passes through. Once the tip of the catheter reaches its destination (the PA), only the PA and PAOP waveforms can be measured.

TAKE HOME POINTS

Postprocedure

- To arrive at the most accurate measurement, record waveforms obtained during insertion on paper for documentation purposes.

⚠️ Be very careful **not** to tighten the sleeve too tight on PA catheter—it may crimp the catheter. Tighten the sleeve just enough to keep the catheter from slipping.

Once acceptable measurements are recorded, the physician will suture the introducer in place and the nurse will perform the following:

- Assist in placing a sterile clear occlusive dressing over the site.
- Securely tape the catheter to the patient's chest to prevent inadvertent dislodgement or migration. The level of centimeter marking on the catheter should be noted. Normal position is 45 to 55 cm.
- Tighten the sterile sleeve around the catheter just enough to keep it from slipping but not enough to occlude it.
- Ensure that a chest x-ray film is ordered to confirm placement and to rule out a pneumothorax, any kinking, or other complications.
- Obtain additional hemodynamic calculations such as CO, cardiac index, and systemic vascular resistance (SVR) (see Chapter 8).
- Continuously monitor and assess waveforms to ensure that the PA catheter remains in the correct position.

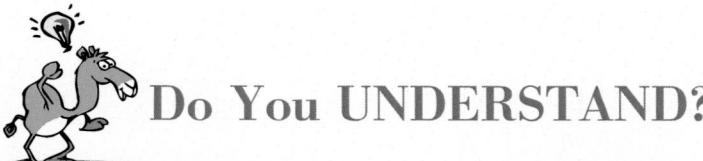

Do You UNDERSTAND?

DIRECTIONS: **Fill in the blanks to complete the following statements.**

1. The PA catheter is marked with black lines to indicate the depth of insertion. These black lines are marked in increments of _____ cm.

2. Hemodynamic measurements such as preload, afterload, and contractility can be obtained by inserting a _____

_____

_____..

3. PA pressure monitoring allows the nurse to measure _____- sided pressures related to the pulmonary circulation and the right side of the heart. It also allows the nurse to *indirectly* measure _____- sided pressures related to the systemic circulation.

DIRECTIONS: **To prepare the monitor for PA catheter insertion, the nurse should perform four steps. Match each action listed in Column A with the correct description in Column B, placing the corresponding letter in the space provided.**

Column A   Column B

_____ 4. Zero   a. The pressure tubing and transducer

_____ 5. Connect   b. The transducer tubing to the monitor cable

_____ 6. Flush   c. The PA distal line on the monitor by opening the stopcock to air

_____ 7. Level   d. The side port of the transducer stopcock with the patient's RA

Answers: 1. 10; 2. pulmonary artery catheter; 3. right, left; 4. c; 5. b; 6. a; 7. d.

DIRECTIONS: Match each of the ports listed in Column A with its use in Column B, and place the corresponding letter in the space provided.

	Column A	Column B
______	8. Distal port	a. Best to infuse dopamine.
______	9. Proximal injectate port	b. Connected to transducer; used to draw mixed venous gases; do not use for infusion.
______	10. Proximal infusion port or VIP	c. Connected to transducer; used to measure CVP and CO.

DIRECTIONS: Identify the following statements as *true* (T) or *false* (F).

______ 11. Informed consent is required for PA catheter insertion.

______ 12. Bedside fluoroscopy is always necessary for PA catheter insertion.

DIRECTIONS: Name two changes in the waveform noted during insertion that confirm that the catheter has passed from the RV through the pulmonic valve.

13. ______________________________

14. ______________________________

DIRECTIONS: Label the following waveform obtained during insertion of a PA catheter.

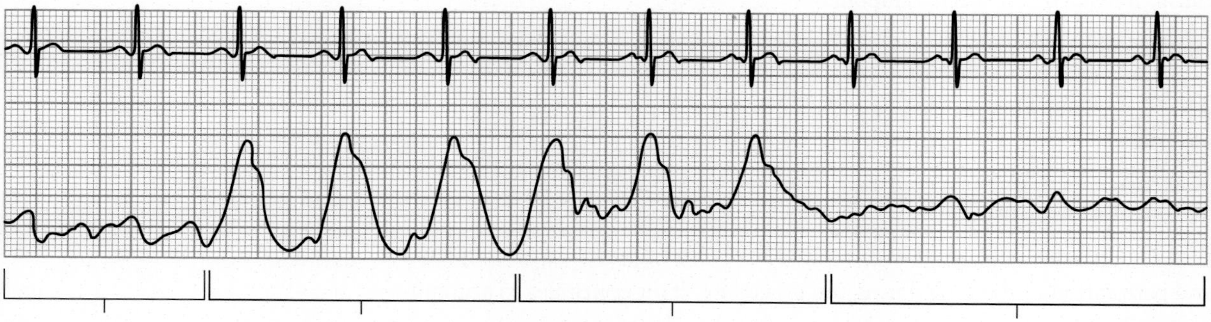

15. __________ 16. __________ 17. __________ 18. __________

Answers: 8. b; 9. c; 10. a; 11. T; 12. F; 13. appearance of dicrotic notch; 14. systolic pressure will be the same but the diastolic pressure will be higher; 15. RA; 16. RV; 17. PA; 18. PAOP or PCWP.

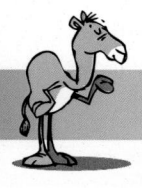

What IS the List of Possible Complications of Pulmonary Artery Catheter Insertion?

During Insertion

Immediate life-threatening complications that may occur during insertion include pneumothorax and venous air embolism. Both of these complications can be rapidly fatal, but both are usually preventable. Other complications that may occur during insertion include dysrhythmias, dislodgement of the catheter wire, or excessive bleeding.

Postinsertion

Complications that may occur within hours to days after insertion include dysrhythmias (especially right bundle branch block or third-degree atrioventricular block), catheter-related infection, catheter dislodgement, thrombophlebitis, and pulmonary rupture. The catheter may migrate into a small arteriole where it persistently wedges itself as it warms and softens to body temperature. It is important to recognize the wedge waveform to identify this complication and pull back the catheter before pulmonary ischemia or infarction occurs. Rarely PA rupture can result from overinflation of the balloon in an already distended arteriole. Other reported but rare complications are intracardiac thrombus or embolus, endocarditis, and ruptured myocardium leading to cardiac tamponade.

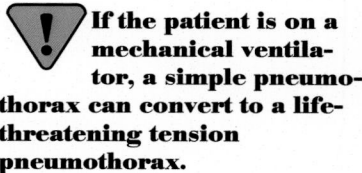

TAKE HOME POINTS

Pneumothorax may occur during the subclavian approach but not when using the femoral approach.

If the patient is on a mechanical ventilator, a simple pneumothorax can convert to a life-threatening tension pneumothorax.

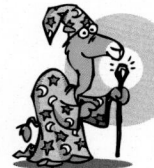

What You NEED TO KNOW

Tension Pneumothorax

A pneumothorax may occur as a result of inadvertent puncture of the pleura and perforation of the lung during the procedure. If air continues to accumulate in the pleural space and cannot escape, a life-threatening tension pneumothorax can occur. Signs of a tension pneumothorax include the following:

- Sudden onset of hypotension
- Respiratory distress
- Unequal breath sounds

- Hyperresonance to percussion
- Tracheal deviation
- Marked increase in peak airway pressure in ventilated patients

Venous Air Embolism

> ⚠ **A pressure gradient of even 4 mm Hg across a 14 gauge catheter may draw approximately 90 ml of air per second into the venous circulation and produce a sudden fatal air embolism.**

A venous air embolism may occur if air enters the central circulation when the introducer needle is open to air. The negative intrathoracic pressure brings the venous pressure below atmospheric pressure, and air flows through the needle to enter the circulation. The air that enters the central veins passes through the right heart chambers and embolizes in the pulmonary circulation. Signs of venous air embolism include the following:

- Sudden onset dyspnea
- Tachypnea
- Chest pain
- Hypotension
- Cardiac arrest

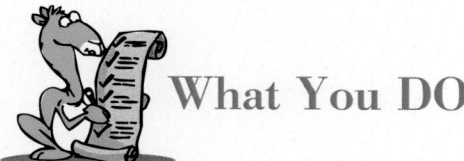 # What You DO

Tension Pneumothorax

Immediate insertion of a percutaneous needle into the second intercostal space at the midclavicular line on the side of the pneumothorax is the treatment for tension pneumothorax. This procedure should be followed with the insertion of a standard chest tube. Only the physician or a credentialed advanced practice nurse performs these procedures.

Venous Air Embolism

If an air embolism is suspected, place the patient on the left side with the head down (air will rise to the RA) while attempting to aspirate the air from the venous catheter. Administer 100% oxygen. Safety measures to prepare against venous air embolism occurrence are the following:

- Prevent hypovolemia.
- Increase the CVP by placing the patient in the Trendelenburg position during insertion.
- Instruct the patient to perform a Valsalva maneuver (bearing down) while the catheter is open to air. This maneuver prevents deep inspiration, which could increase the risk of air entry.
- Place a sterile gloved thumb over the open hub to prevent air entry.

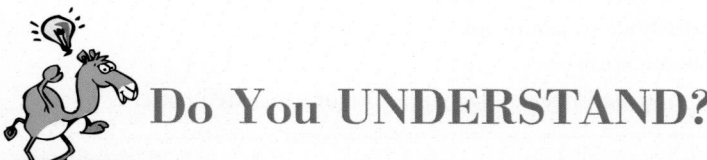

Do You UNDERSTAND?

DIRECTIONS: **Fill in the blanks to complete each of the following statements.**

1. _____ and _____ _____

_____ are life-threatening complications that can

occur during PA catheter insertion.

2. A _____ _____ can occur if the bal-

loon is left inflated too long.

CHAPTER

7 Pulmonary Artery Pressures and Waveforms

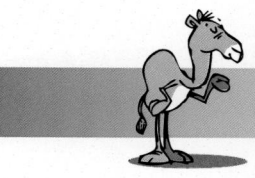

What IS Pulmonary Artery Pressure Monitoring?

Pressures within the lungs (right-sided pressures) are normally much lower than those in the systemic circulation (left-sided pressures). The following two reasons explain this:

1. Because the lungs are located in close proximity to the heart, the right ventricle (RV) does not have to generate a high level of pressure to pump blood such a short distance. The left ventricle (LV), on the other hand, has to generate a significantly greater level of pressure to pump blood all the way from the head to the toes.

2. The low pressure in the pulmonary system is critical to accommodate adequate gas exchange in the lungs. If the pressure in the pulmonary capillaries is too high, then intravascular fluid is forced into the alveoli, resulting in interference with the oxygen and carbon dioxide exchange and causing pulmonary edema.

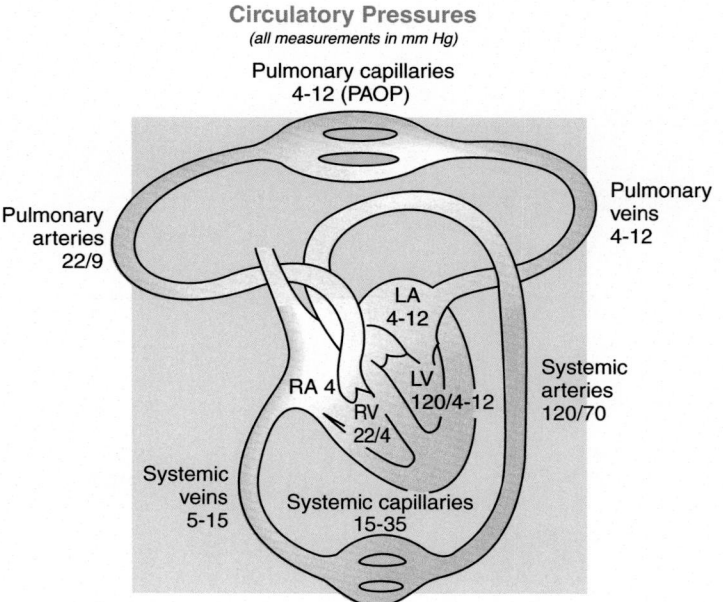

Circulatory Pressures
(all measurements in mm Hg)

Pulmonary capillaries
4-12 (PAOP)

Pulmonary arteries
22/9

Pulmonary veins
4-12

LA
4-12

RA 4

LV
120/4-12

Systemic arteries
120/70

RV
22/4

Systemic veins
5-15

Systemic capillaries
15-35

The pulmonary artery (PA) pressure waveform has the same characteristics as the arterial waveform, except with lower pressures. Note the following scale. This example would be interpreted as a PAP of 31/13 mm Hg.

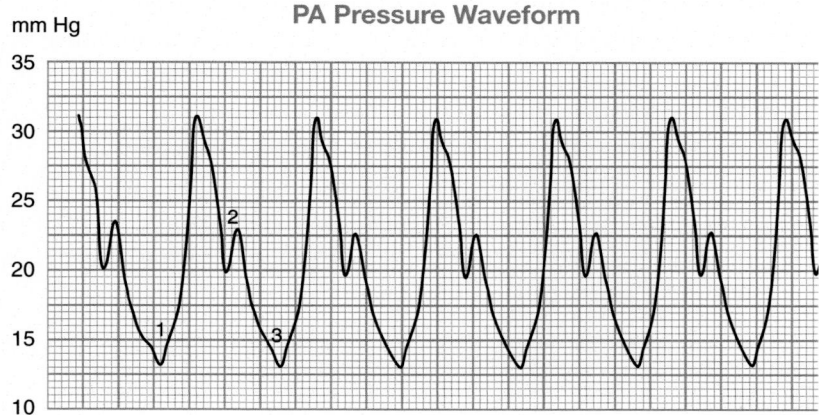

PA Pressure Waveform

mm Hg

1 = Sharp upstroke

1. Sharp upstroke (systolic ejection into pulmonary artery)
2. Dicrotic notch (closure of pulmonic valve)
3. Gradual downslope (end-diastole and opening of pulmonic valve)

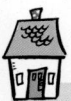

TAKE HOME POINTS

The nurse should be sure to use the correct scale on the monitor for the PA range. A 0 to 40 scale is acceptable unless the PA pressures are unusually high. If the wrong scale is used, then the waveform is difficult to interpret.

However, in the PA pressure waveform, the dicrotic notch represents closure of the pulmonic valve (rather than the aortic valve), and end diastole (gradual downslope) represents the opening of the pulmonic valve (rather than the aortic valve). Careful attention should always be paid to the scale on the left side of the monitor to distinguish whether the wave is a systemic arterial waveform or a pulmonary arterial waveform.

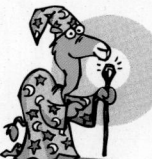

What You NEED TO KNOW

Pulmonary Arterial Pressures

Once the PA catheter is inserted, it continuously measures the pulmonary artery systolic (PAS) and pulmonary artery diastolic (PAD) pressures. The pulmonary arterial systolic (PAS) pressure is the amount of pressure necessary to open the pulmonary valve and eject blood into the pulmonary circulation. The PAS is the same as the RV pressure when the pulmonic valve is open. Normal PAS pressure is approximately 15 to 30 mm Hg with a mean pressure of 22 mm Hg. The PAD pressure is the amount of resistance in the lungs (pulmonary vascular resistance [PVR]) in between heartbeats. The PAD reflects pressure in the pulmonary vasculature when the pulmonic valve is closed and the tricuspid valve is open. Normal PAD pressure is 6 to 12 mm Hg with a mean pressure of 9 mm Hg. It is higher than the RV diastolic pressure because of the gradient created when the pulmonic valve closes. To summarize, the average PA pressure is approximately 22 mm Hg systolic, 9 mm Hg diastolic.

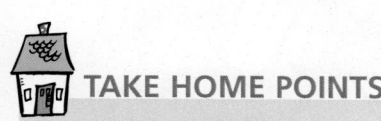

TAKE HOME POINTS

PA pressures are *right-sided* pressures.

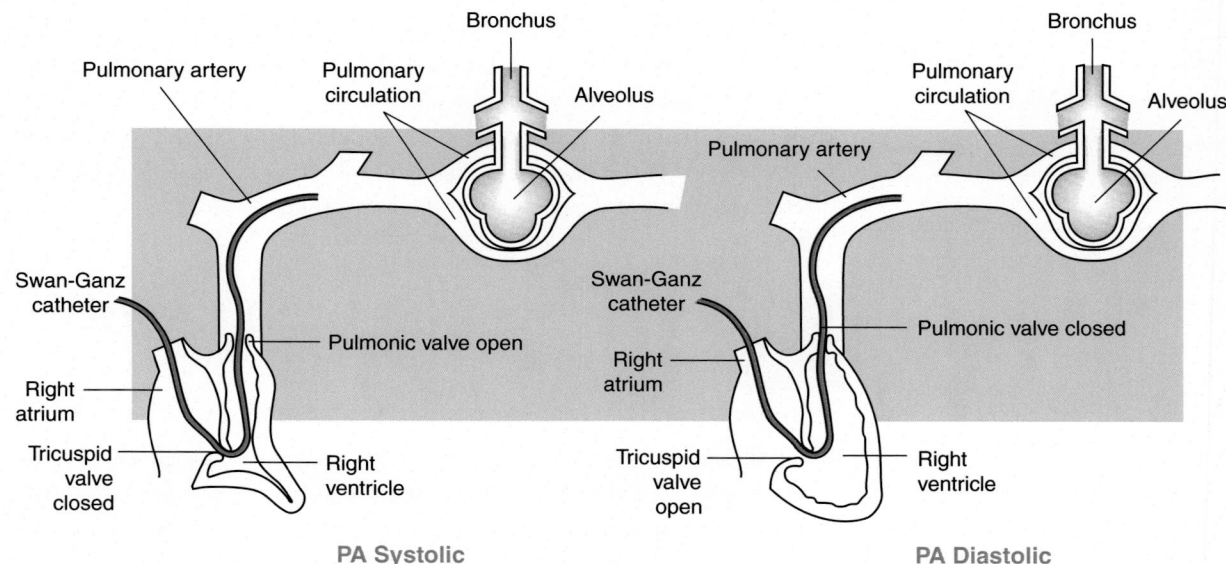

PA Systolic   **PA Diastolic**

Right Atrial and Right Ventricular Pressures

Before the PA catheter reaches the PA, it must pass through the right atrium (RA) and RV. (See Chapter 5 for a review of RA or central venous pressure [CVP].) RV pressures are higher than RA pressures because the RV must generate enough pressure to open the pulmonic valve (RV systolic pressure).

The pulmonic valve snaps shut during diastole, and the tricuspid valve opens to allow ventricular filling. During this time, RV diastolic pressure is equal to the RA pressure, because the valve between the two is open. Normal RV systolic pressure is 15 to 30 mm Hg (the same as PAS). Normal RV diastolic pressure is 0 to 8 mm Hg (the same as the RA pressure or CVP). In summary, an average RV pressure might be somewhere in the middle of each, or approximately 22 mm Hg systolic over 4 mm Hg diastolic.

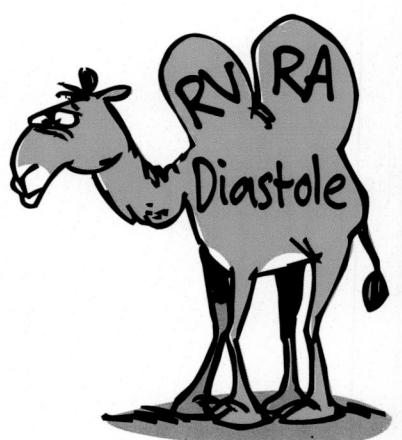

Right Ventricular and Pulmonary Artery Pressure

RV systolic and PAS pressures should be equal. During systole the pulmonic valve is open and blood is ejected into the PA. During the split second while the valve is open, the pressures on either side of the valve become equal, as if the valve were not there. The same action happens on the left side of the heart. The aortic valve opens and blood is ejected into the aorta; during this time while the aortic valve is open, the LV systolic pressure equals the systolic aortic arterial pressure.

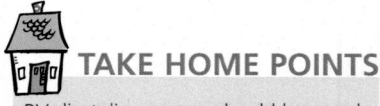

TAKE HOME POINTS

RV diastolic pressure should be equal to the RA mean pressure.

However, when the valves close during diastole, a separation between the two chambers exists, and the pressure in the vessel being measured is no longer related to the pressure of the chamber on the other side of the valve. The pressure in the vessel being measured is solely dependent on its own internal pressures. Normal RV diastolic pressure is 0 to 8 mm Hg. Normal PAD pressure is 6 to 12 mm Hg. The level is higher as a result of the resistance of the blood vessels in the lungs (PVR). In the systemic circulation, it is called *systemic vascular resistance* (SVR).

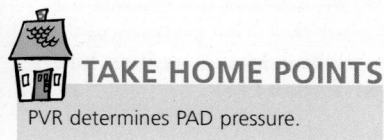

TAKE HOME POINTS

PVR determines PAD pressure.

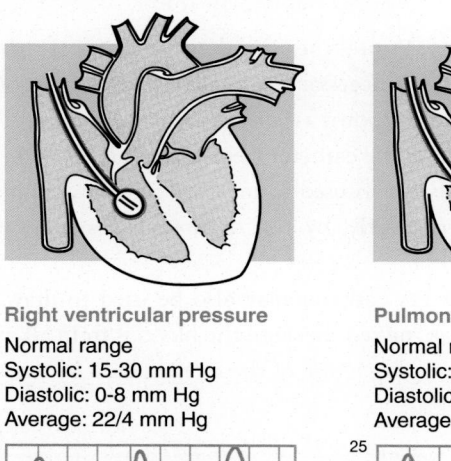

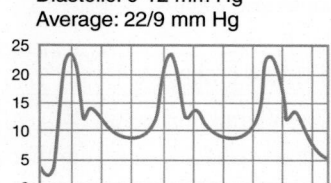

Right ventricular pressure
Normal range
Systolic: 15-30 mm Hg
Diastolic: 0-8 mm Hg
Average: 22/4 mm Hg

Pulmonary artery pressure
Normal range
Systolic: 15-30 mm Hg
Diastolic: 6-12 mm Hg
Average: 22/9 mm Hg

Assessment of Pulmonary Arterial Systolic and Diastolic Pressures

PAS and PAD pressures reflect right-sided pressures. If elevated, this indicates a lung problem. Assessment of PA pressures can help distinguish between primary lung problems and lung problems caused by the heart.

Because PAS pressure is equal to RV systolic pressure, the PAS pressure is high whenever the RV has to generate a higher pressure to open the pulmonic valve. PAS pressure must be high enough to overcome PAD pressure. Pulmonary diastolic pressure increases whenever the blood vessels in the lungs are constricted (increased PVR). Any condition that causes increased PVR will increase both pulmonary systolic and diastolic pressures. This occurs in pulmonary hypertension, chronic hypoxemia, and pulmonary embolus. Chronic hypoxemia may be the result of many conditions, including chronic obstructive pulmonary disease (COPD) and sleep apnea.

PVR is considered the *afterload* for the RV. It elevates when the pulmonary vessels are constricted. The RV and PAS pressures must elevate to work against this resistance. Blood backs up into the lungs, which causes further increased resistance to RV pumping. For example, a PA pressure, which rises to 65 mm Hg systolic and 35 mm Hg diastolic, indicates pulmonary hypertension. Low PA pressures, similar to systemic pressures, are usually related to low-volume status.

Other Uses for a Pulmonary Artery Catheter

1. Besides measurement of PA pressures and determination of right-sided pressures, the PA catheter is necessary to obtain pulmonary artery occlusion pressure (PAOP) (also known as left ventricular end–diastolic pressure [LVEDP]) by wedging the catheter (see section on PAOP).
2. The proximal injectate port is used to measure cardiac output, either continuously or intermittently, by the thermodilution method (see Chapter 8).
3. The distal port of the PA catheter may also be used to draw mixed venous blood gases. It is "mixed" because the blood is from all over the body and reflects an overall picture of the oxygen used by the various tissues and organs.

MIXED VENOUS BLOOD SAMPLING

- Ensure that the balloon is deflated.
- Observe waveform to ensure that catheter is not in the PAOP position.
- Aspirate from the PA distal port 3 to 5 ml of blood slowly and discard.
- Aspirate the test sample slowly.
- Avoid rapid withdrawal of blood, because this may cause oxygenated blood from the pulmonary capillaries to be drawn into the syringe, falsely elevating the mixed venous SvO_2.

---

4. Some PA catheters can measure continuous venous oxygen saturation (SvO_2). A special adapter is needed to take advantage of this feature (refer to Chapter 9).
5. Some catheters have an additional pacer port that can pace either the atria or the ventricles.
6. Some newer ejection fraction catheters allow the calculation of right ventricular end–systolic pressure (RVESP) and right ventricular end–diastolic pressure (RVEDP), as well as the standard features.

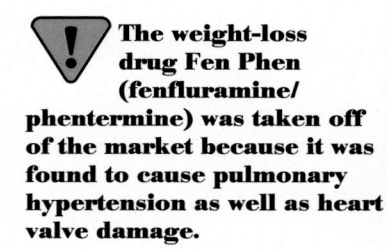

The weight-loss drug Fen Phen (fenfluramine/ phentermine) was taken off of the market because it was found to cause pulmonary hypertension as well as heart valve damage.

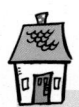

TAKE HOME POINTS

- Most right-sided heart failure is due to left-sided heart failure.
- Pure right-sided heart failure that is **NOT** due to left-sided heart failure is called *cor pulmonale*.
- Any condition which causes increased PVR will cause an increase in pulmonary systolic and diastolic pressures. Examples include pulmonary hypertension, chronic hypoxemia, and pulmonary embolus.

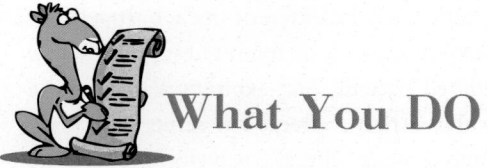

What You DO

How to Measure Pulmonary Artery Pressures

Once inserted, when the catheter tip is resting in the PA, between wedgings, a waveform will be created by the electronic monitor. The electronic monitor will average the last few seconds of waveforms and provide a digital printout. This waveform may vary with respiration. Therefore it is usually best not to use this printout because it is averaging the peaks and valleys of respiratory artifact. The measurement should be taken at the end of expiration when the lungs are quiet to get a true reading.

In a spontaneously breathing patient, intrapulmonary pressures will decrease slightly on inspiration and increase on expiration. In a mechanically ventilated patient, intrapulmonary pressures will increase on inspiration and decrease on expiration.

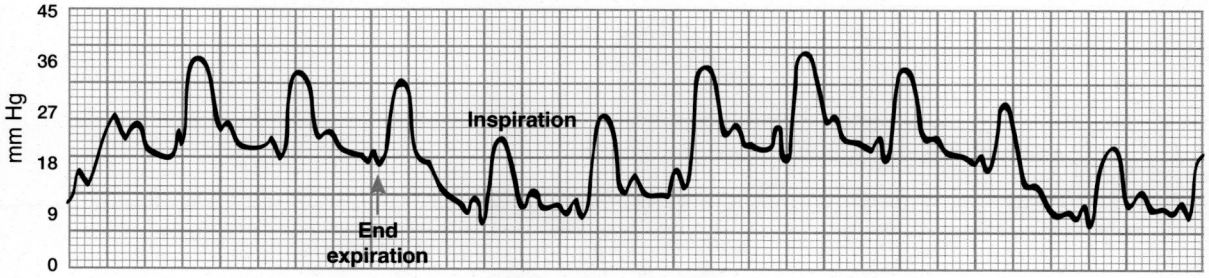

Spontaneous Ventilation

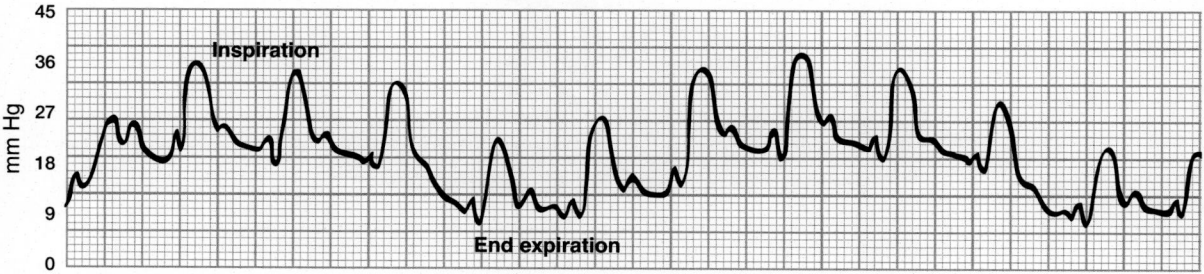

Mechanical Ventilation

Therefore the point of end-expiration will be different in each. In a spontaneously breathing patient, end-expiration will be the highest point before the dip. In a mechanically ventilated patient, end-expiration will be the lowest point before the rise. It is always best to freeze the screen and print the recording on paper to have time to work with the waveform for a more accurate measurement and for documentation purposes.

Elevated PA pressures occur in pulmonary hypertension, chronic pulmonary disease, mitral valve disease, LV failure, hypoxemia, and pulmonary emboli. Below-normal PA pressures occur primarily in conditions that produce hypovolemia.

Troubleshooting

Technical errors may occur in leveling or zeroing and can give inaccurate results.

If the transducer is too high, it can give a false low reading. If too low, it can give a false high reading. Respiratory variation can cause alterations in interpretation of waveforms. The nurse should always measure PA pressure at end-expiration. (Refer to Chapter 3 for a review of transducer setup.)

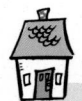

TAKE HOME POINTS

- To remember when to take the end-expiration reading on a mechanically ventilated patient, the nurse should use the mnemonic "Valley = Ventilator."
- Remember, normal PAS and PAD pressures are approximately 22/9 mm Hg.
- PA pressure readings should always be taken at end-expiration.

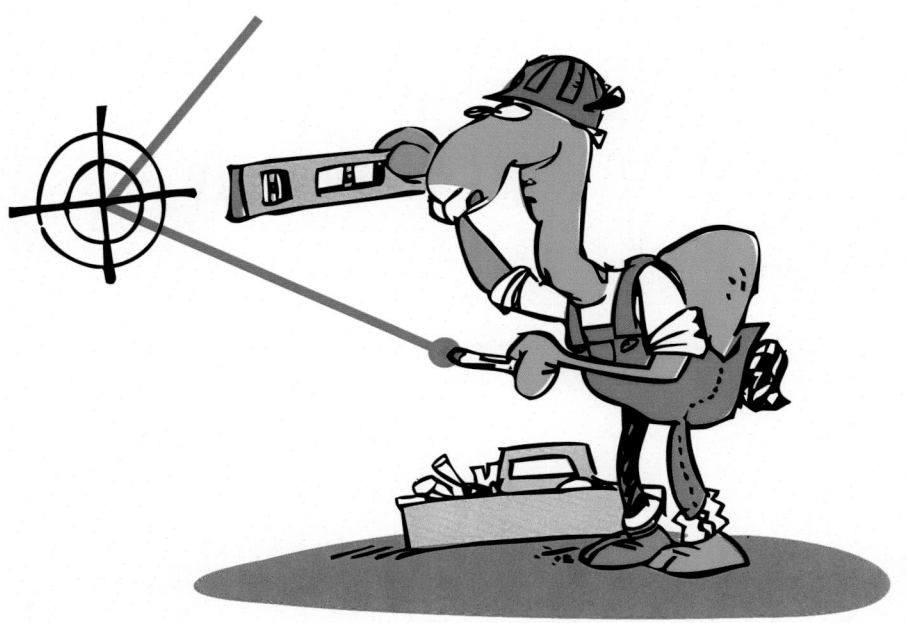

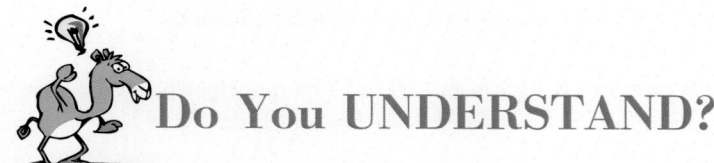

Do You UNDERSTAND?

DIRECTIONS: Circle the correct word(s) to complete the following statements.

1. When the pulmonic valve is open, RV and PA pressures should be **equal/unequal.** This is during **systole/diastole.**

2. When the pulmonic valve is closed, RV and PA pressures should be **equal/unequal.** This is during **systole/diastole.**

3. The pulmonary blood flow system is normally a **high/low** pressure system.

DIRECTIONS: Match each statement in Column A with an answer in Column B.

Column A	Column B
_____ 4. Normal RA pressure (mean)	a. 22/4 mm Hg
_____ 5. Normal RV pressure	b. 0 to 8 mm Hg

DIRECTIONS: Fill in the blanks to complete each of the following statements.

6. Normal PAS pressure is _____ – _____ mm Hg.

7. Normal PAD pressure is _____ – _____ mm Hg.

8. A pulmonary pressure of 65/35 mm Hg would represent

_____ _____.

9. When the PA catheter is **NOT** wedged, it is continuously monitoring

the _____ and _____ pressures.

DIRECTIONS: **Provide answers to the following questions.**

10. If the PA pressure changes from 25/12 to 25/4 mm Hg, what is the most likely cause?

_____

_____

11. Is the following waveform a PA or arterial waveform? Hint: Look at the scale. What is the interpretation?

_____ _____ mm Hg

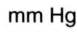

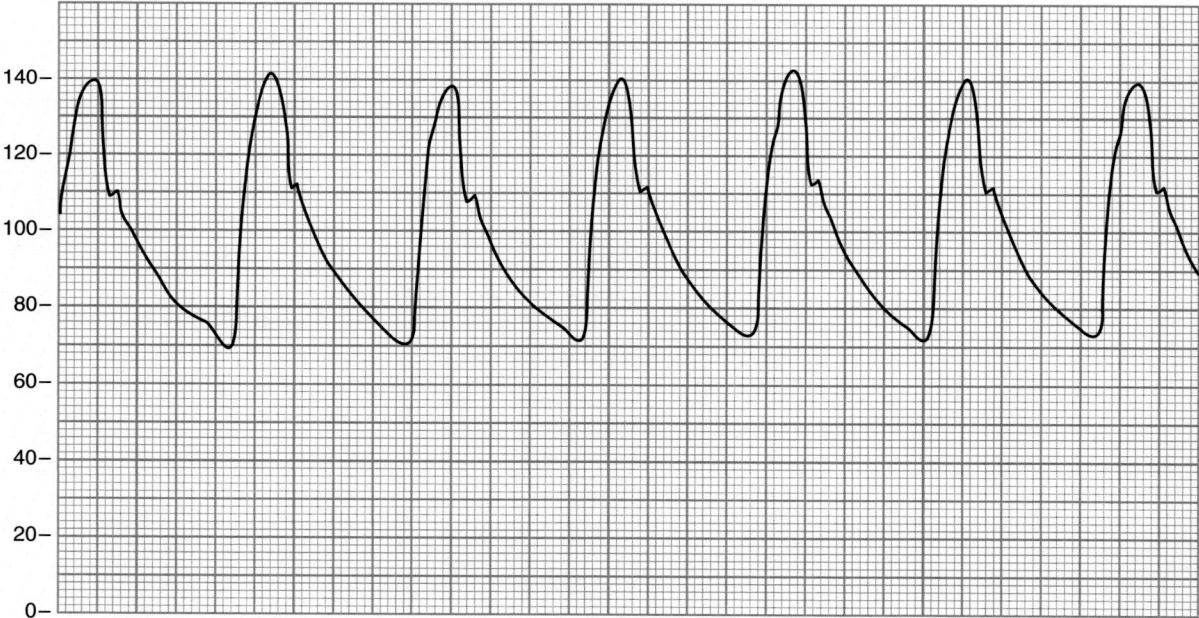

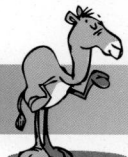

What IS Preload?

Preload is the amount of fluid in the LV at the end of diastole that stretches the fibers and determines the amount of blood that is pumped out with the next systole. The nurse should remember that preload is one of the determinants of stroke volume (SV) and therefore cardiac output. It is used clinically to assess LV function and systemic fluid status. In most acute settings, it is considered more important to assess the left side of the heart than the right.

Preload is measured by obtaining the PAOP, which is also called the *pulmonary arterial wedge pressure* (PAWP) or the *pulmonary capillary wedge pressure* (PCWP). The PAOP is an indirect measurement of pulmonary venous pressure. More importantly, it also reflects left atrial (LA) pressure, and indirectly, LVEDP.

Normal PAOP range is 6 to 12 mm Hg. Such a narrow range exists between the systolic and the diastolic pressure that an average or mean is used (just like in CVP measurement). In general, low values reflect hypovolemia or may be the result of vasodilator drugs. High values indicate hypervolemia or LV failure, ischemia, or constrictive pericarditis. Mitral valve abnormalities will also cause elevations in PAOP.

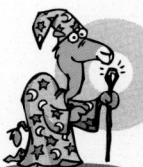

What You NEED TO KNOW

What Pulmonary Artery Occlusion Pressure Measures

When the PA catheter is not being wedged (sitting in the PA in between wedging), it is measuring the PA (right-sided) pressures. Once it is wedged, the catheter is measuring back pressure from the left side of the heart. The number obtained while wedging is known as the *PAOP*, which should be equivalent to the LA pressure and the LVEDP or *preload.*

Preload is important because, as a determinant of SV, it indicates how much volume the heart has to pump. Too much preload means too much volume, and this can cause fluid to back up and cause symptoms of heart failure. Too little preload means too little volume, and this can cause the heart not to stretch enough to elicit a strong contraction. (Refer to Chapter 2 to review information on the Frank-Starling curve.)

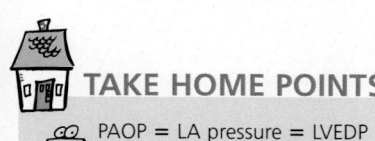

TAKE HOME POINTS

PAOP = LA pressure = LVEDP
= LV preload = PCWP = PAWP

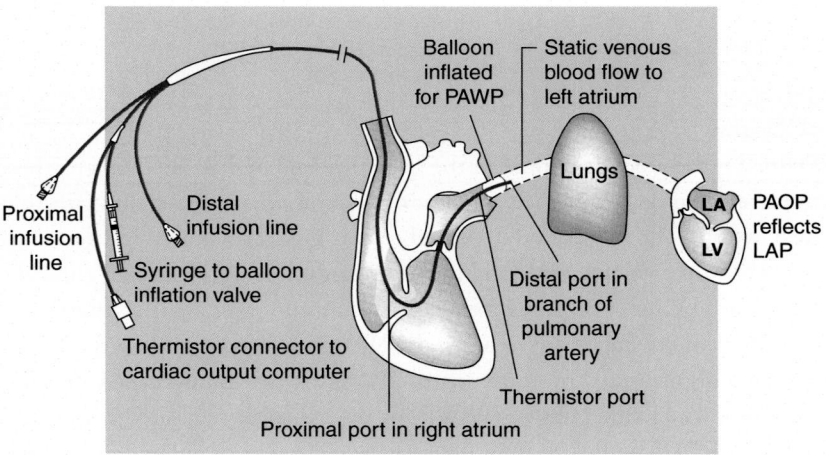

Why Pulmonary Artery Occlusion Pressure is Measured

Hemodynamic monitoring can detect early changes in SV in the patient before symptoms occur. The determinants of SV are preload, afterload, and contractility. The wedge pressure measures LV preload. LV preload is not exactly the same as RV preload, so the CVP (RV preload) cannot be used as a measurement of LV function. By the time the CVP increases, the patient may already have signs of volume overload.

One of the main situations in which a PAOP is useful is in hypotension. Blood pressure (BP) may drop for four reasons: (1) the heart rate is too fast, (2) the heart rate is too slow, (3) the SV may be inadequate, or (4) there may be a combination of these problems. The SV may be inadequate either because of inadequate volume (preload), too much resistance to pumping (afterload), or poor pumping ability of the heart (contractility). When trying to differentiate between the causes of decreased SV, PAOP should be ruled out first. Then the other two parameters should be examined.

Pulmonary Artery Occlusion Pressure Waveform

The characteristics and interpretation of PAOP (LA) and CVP (RA) waveforms are similar. The difference between interpreting a CVP and a PAOP waveform mainly centers on the delay in waveform correlation with the electrocardiogram (ECG). This delay is based on the distance from the tip of the PA catheter to the LA. For example, the *a* wave starts near the end of the QRS complex on a PAOP waveform. The process of averaging the *a* wave's highest and lowest values is the same as previously described for CVP readings. The PAOP should be approximately equal to or 2 to 4 mm Hg less than the PAD pressure.

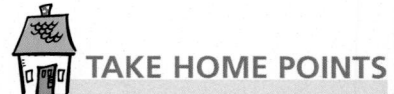
TAKE HOME POINTS

- The *a* and *v* waves in the PAOP waveform relate to the **LA**.
- The *a* and *v* waves in the CVP waveform relate to the **RA**.
- Large *a* waves are seen when the left atrium contracts against a closed mitral valve.
- Large *v* waves are seen during mitral valve insufficiency and left heart failure.

How Pulmonary Artery Diastolic Pressure Relates to Pulmonary Artery Occlusion Pressure

During diastole, the

$$LVEDP = LA\ pressure = PV\ pressure = PAOP$$

This is because a measurement from an obstructed pulmonary capillary will reflect an uninterrupted flow of blood to the LA, because no valves exist in the PA system. Therefore the PAD pressure should correlate closely with or be slightly higher than the PAOP. PA pressure must be high enough to ensure blood flow through the lungs to the LA. Therefore the mean PA pressure must always be higher than the LA pressure (PAOP), or else blood flow through the lungs will stop. If the PAD value is less than the LA or PAOP, either a very low pulmonary blood flow state exists or the waveforms have been misinterpreted (usually caused by overwedging).

The PAOP may be several mm Hg lower than the PAD pressure. Certain pathologic conditions such as tachycardia, hypoxia, and pulmonary disease may prevent these pressures from correlating. Mitral regurgitation may also cause the PAOP to appear higher than it is because of the large v waves. It is important to recognize whether a correlation exists within 4 mm Hg; if it does, it is not necessary to wedge the catheter as frequently. It is assumed that when the mitral valve is open, LA pressure reflects LVEDP. This is true as long as no mitral valve disease is present. Mitral regurgitation causes reflux into the LA, which can increase LA and pulmonary venous pressure, but does not necessarily reflect LVEDP. Mitral stenosis also can increase LA and pulmonary venous pressure but not necessarily reflect LVEDP.

The wedge pressure is not a benign procedure; it could cause PA rupture, especially in pulmonary hypertension when the vessels are distended and friable. Therefore the PAD reading should be substituted for PAOP whenever possible. The PAD value may not be used for the PAOP in the cases of pulmonary embolus, chronic hypoxemia (as in COPD), tachycardia, mitral valve disease, and cor pulmonale.

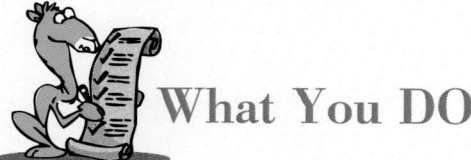

What You DO

A PAOP is obtained from the distal port of the PA catheter when the balloon on the catheter is inflated. The catheter will advance along with the blood flow and enter a smaller branch of the arteriole where it will occlude

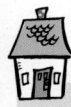

TAKE HOME POINTS

The PAOP should never exceed the wedge pressure. If it does, the cause is usually technical—e.g., overwedging.

TAKE HOME POINTS

- The PAD should be used as a substitute for the PAOP whenever possible—ESPECIALLY if the patient has pulmonary hypertension.
- Digital displays may be unreliable if a lot of respiratory variation exists. It is best to use the strip recorder for waveform analysis.

- **PA catheter wedging has the potential for rupturing the PA.**
As long as the PAD is within 4 mm Hg of the PAOP, it is acceptable to use the PAD as an indicator of LVEDP without having to wedge the catheter.
- **Should hemoptysis occur after wedging, the PA catheter should be pulled back and the patient intubated and placed on positive end–expiratory pressure (PEEP). Bronchoscopy is performed unless hemothorax is present with unstable hemodynamics, in which case an emergency thoracotomy should be performed.**

the distal blood flow and become wedged. At this point the catheter is measuring backflow from the left side of the heart. The wedge pressure (PAOP) is really the same as the LA pressure in most patients, because no valves or pressure gradients exist between the two. The frequency of wedging will be dictated by the physician and by hospital policy.

Inflation of the balloon is performed only for a few seconds to avoid a disruption in pulmonary blood flow. It should only be inflated to the volume necessary to obtain the PAOP waveform.

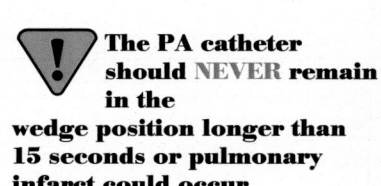

The PA catheter should NEVER remain in the wedge position longer than 15 seconds or pulmonary infarct could occur.

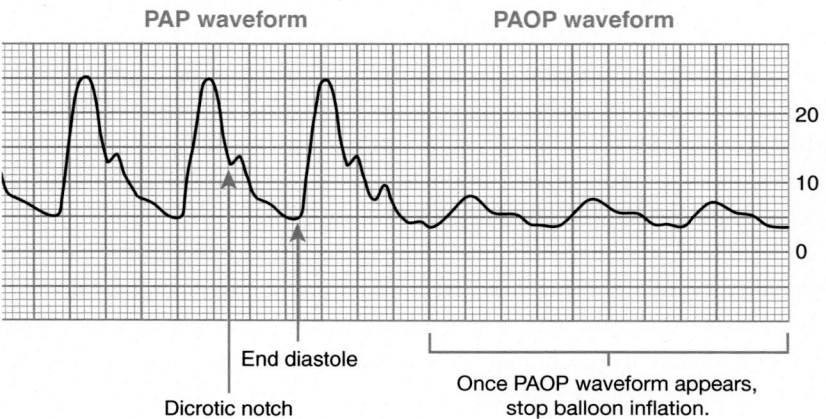

PAP waveform   PAOP waveform

20
10
0

End diastole

Dicrotic notch

Once PAOP waveform appears, stop balloon inflation.

TAKE HOME POINTS

The nurse should be sure to use the correct scale on the monitor when wedging. The 0-40 mm Hg scale is acceptable unless the PA pressures are unusually high. If the wrong scale is used, the waveform will be difficult to interpret.

The nurse should notice how much air it takes to inflate the balloon; it should not be inflated longer than 15 seconds. The air should be allowed to passively escape from the syringe, and care should be taken to avoid aspiration. Forceful aspiration can damage the balloon. The PAOP waveform can be "frozen" on the monitor screen and hemodynamic calculations obtained after wedging. Just as in PA measurements, the PAOP (PAWP) measurement should be obtained at end-expiration. This does not mean that the nurse has to "catch" the patient during this phase of respiration and inflate at precisely the right time. It means that he or she needs to recognize respiratory variation on the monitor and its relationship to whether the patient is breathing spontaneously or mechanically ventilated.

The PAOP in the previous figure is easy to interpret because not much respiratory variation exists. The PAOP is 7 to 8 mm Hg. The digital print-out in this patient is likely to be accurate, as opposed to the waveform in the following figure:

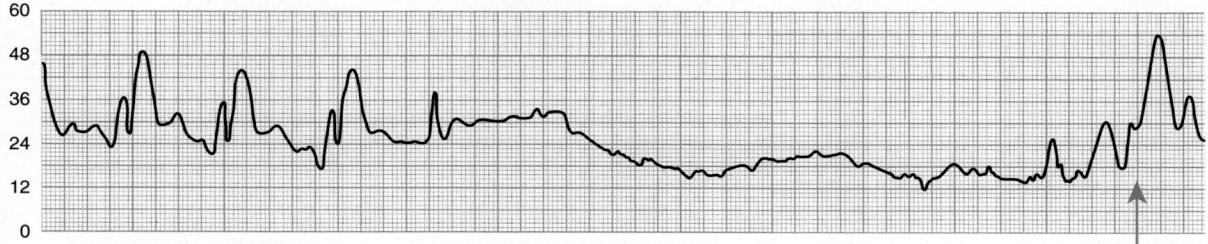

Return of PA waveform after wedging

 The nurse should always ensure that a clearly defined PA pressure returns after wedging.

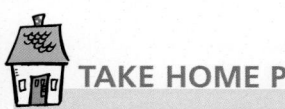 **TAKE HOME POINTS**

- When deflating the balloon, air should be allowed to leave it passively. Actively aspirating the air out of the balloon damages the balloon and is not necessary for complete emptying of the balloon.
- The 1½-ml syringe supplied with the catheter should always be used. The balloon should not be inflated with greater than 1½ ml air. The balloon may rupture.

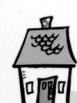 **TAKE HOME POINTS**

Treatment of decreased preload includes administration of intravenous (IV) fluids.

Treatment

The goal of therapy is to maximize cardiac output and oxygen delivery, as well as to prevent or treat pulmonary edema. An elevated preload can lead to symptoms of heart failure. Therapy for increased preload is aimed at decreasing venous return. The most obvious way to decrease preload is to give diuretics to "unload" fluid from the body and therefore decrease the workload of the heart. Another way to decrease preload is by the administration of venous vasodilators, which cause venous pooling of blood. The venules (small, terminal portions of veins) are capacitance vessels, which means that they swell or shrink depending on the amount of volume they hold. They do not constrict and dilate like arteries. By swelling or dilating with blood in the extremities, the fluid is prevented from returning to the heart and therefore the workload of the heart is decreased. Examples of drugs that cause venous dilation and pooling include nitroglycerin, morphine sulfate, and nesiritide.

Patient Education

Patients requiring hemodynamic monitoring are often facing acute life-threatening illness and are typically overwhelmed with anxiety. Not only is there a threat to their physical health but also the intensive care unit (ICU) environment, with all of its monitors, beeps, alarms, and equipment, can cause a sense of helplessness and fear. It is essential to care for the patient's emotional, psychologic, and spiritual needs, in addition to the physical ones. The nurse must connect with the patient, not just the machines. Upon entering a patient's room, the nurse should:

- Identify himself or herself and speak in a nonhurried fashion directly to the patient.

- Establish direct eye contact with the patient before focusing on the IVs or the monitors.
- Take the patient's hand or touch the patient in some way to let the patient know that the nurse is listening.
- Listen seriously to any concerns the patient may have. The issues that concern patients are often quite different from those that concern the nurse.
- Establish a mode of communication with intubated patients who cannot speak.
- Always tell the patient what is being done, and keep the patient and family well-informed about plans for the day (tests, surgery) and any updates or changes to the plan of care.

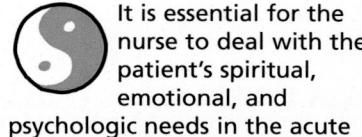

It is essential for the nurse to deal with the patient's spiritual, emotional, and psychologic needs in the acute care environment.

Troubleshooting

Catheter Migration

After the catheter is inserted, the distal tip warms up to body temperature and becomes as soft as cooked spaghetti. It may tend to migrate with the blood flow either farther in or out of the PA.

- If it takes less air to obtain a PAOP value than at a previous inflation, or if an inadvertent wedge waveform is noted on the monitor, the catheter might have migrated further into the PA. It is necessary to immediately pull back the catheter gently through the sleeve until the PA waveform rather than the wedge is displayed. Otherwise a pulmonary infarct may occur.
- If it takes more air to obtain a PAOP, then the catheter might have to be moved to a more proximal location in the PA. If no resistance is felt when the balloon is inflated and no PAOP tracing occurs, then the physician should be notified of a possible balloon rupture and the attempt at inflation should not be continued.
- If resistance is felt but the catheter will not wedge at all, the catheter tip may have moved back even further into the RV. The nurse should look for the characteristic RV waveform. Premature ventricular contractions (PVCs) may also appear. A chest radiograph is usually ordered to confirm placement. Hospital policy dictates whether the nurse can pull back or advance a PA catheter that has migrated in or out of the PA. He or she should notify the physician to readvance the catheter.

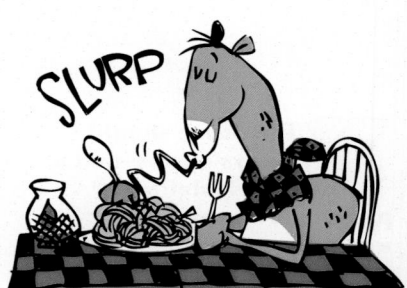

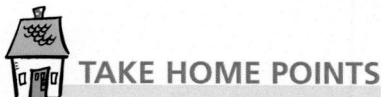

TAKE HOME POINTS

The nurse should always note the centimeter marking on the external portion of the catheter to help judge whether the catheter has migrated in or out. It is marked in 10-cm increments.

Other Troubleshooting Tips

- Digital displays may be unreliable because respiratory variation is counted in averaging. A strip recorder should be used for waveform analysis.
- Overinflation of the balloon tip may cause overwedging. It should be deflated and reinflated with less air.

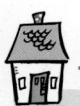

- Technical difficulties such as incorrect catheter or transducer placement, improper zeroing or leveling, or incorrect calibration can interfere with the accuracy of the readings.
- It is acceptable to perform readings with the head of the bed up to a level of 45 degrees. Any higher may make the readings inaccurate.
- Application of PEEP may increase PA pressures, especially in levels of PEEP greater than 15 cm H_2O. This is caused by the increase in PVR. In PEEP greater than 15 cm H_2O, neither PAOP nor the LA pressure accurately reflect the LVEDP.
- Respiratory variation can greatly affect readings. Wedge pressure measurements should be obtained at end-expiration. The appearance of end-expiration will differ depending on whether the patient is spontaneously breathing or being assisted with mechanical ventilation.
- In the spontaneously breathing patient, inspiration causes intrathoracic pressure to decrease, so the lowest points are discounted. The nurse should measure immediately before the pressure dips down. In this example, the digital readout would average all pressures at 14 to 15 mm Hg, which is inaccurate. The end-expiratory value is actually 22 mm Hg. This could make a big difference in the treatment of the patient.

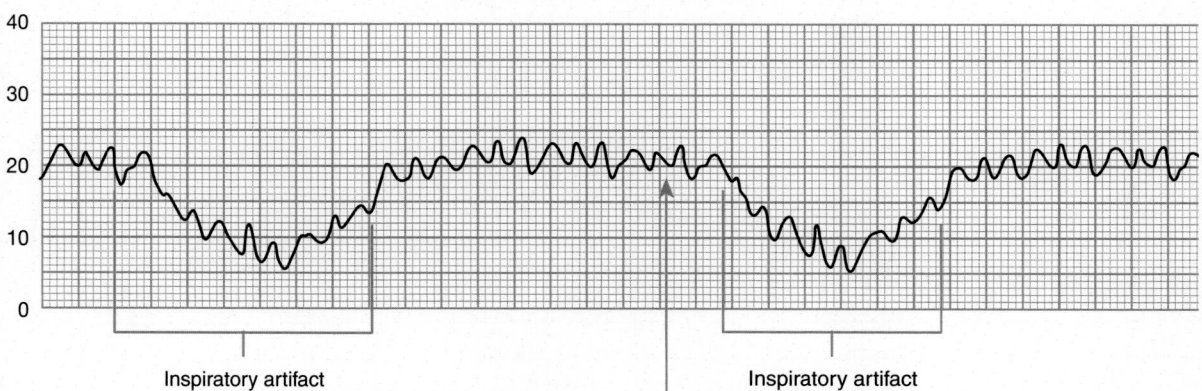

Inspiratory artifact   Inspiratory artifact

End-expiratory points for reading values (mean PAOP = 22 mm Hg)

- Mechanical ventilation can alter the relationship of the waveform to the respiratory cycle. In mechanical ventilation, inspiration causes a positive intrathoracic pressure. Measure immediately before the pressure goes up at end-expiration (the opposite of the above example).
- During wedging for measurement of PAOP, if the catheter "feels" wedged but does not "look" wedged, it may be so because of large *v* waves of mitral regurgitation.

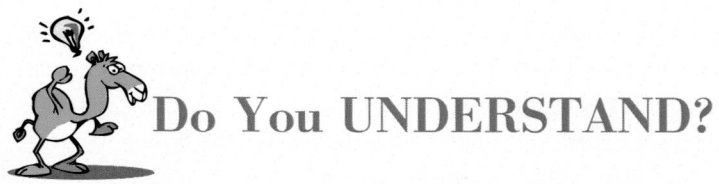

Do You UNDERSTAND?

DIRECTIONS: **Circle the correct response(s).**

1. What are two different names for the volume of blood in the LV immediately before systole? (*preload, LVEDP, afterload*)
2. The preload or LVEDP is measured clinically with a PA catheter by
   obtaining what kind of pressure? (*wedge or PAOP, SVR, MAP*)
3. Treatment of a low preload (PAOP) is to give volume. (*true, false*)

DIRECTIONS: **Fill in the blank to complete the following statement.**

4. An elevated PAOP with large *v* waves may be found in patients with
   what? The catheter "feels" wedged but does not look wedged.

_____

DIRECTIONS: **Select the best answer and place the corresponding
letter in the space provided.**

_____ 5. Upon wedging, the following overwedging waveform is noted.

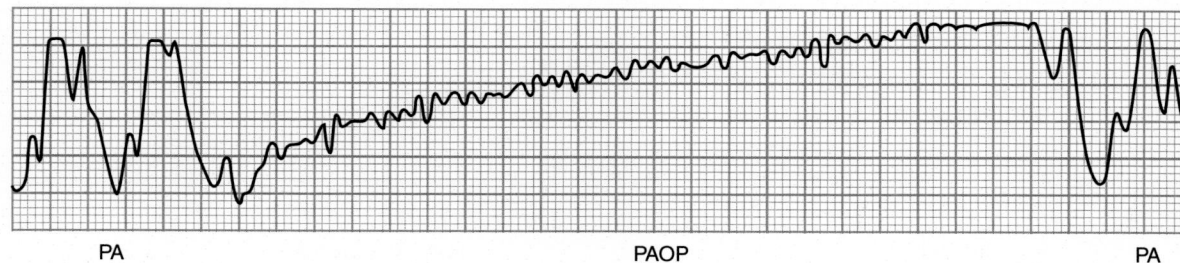

PA   PAOP   PA

What action would you take?
a. Passively allow air to escape from the balloon and rewedge
   with less air.
b. Notify the physician immediately.
c. Flush the catheter.
d. Make sure the balloon is deflated, and gently pull back until
   a PA waveform is resumed.

Answers: 1. preload, LVEDP; 2. wedge or PAOP; 3. true; 4. mitral regurgitation; 5. a.

CO Measurements & Hemodynamic Calculations

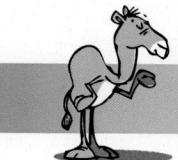

What IS Cardiac Output?

Cardiac output (CO) is the amount of blood pumped out of the heart per minute and is measured in liters per minute. It is determined by two factors: (1) heart rate (HR) and (2) stroke volume (SV). In turn, the determinants of SV are preload, afterload, and contractility. The pulmonary artery (PA) catheter can help determine which of these parameters—preload, afterload, or contractility—may need to be adjusted to optimize CO.

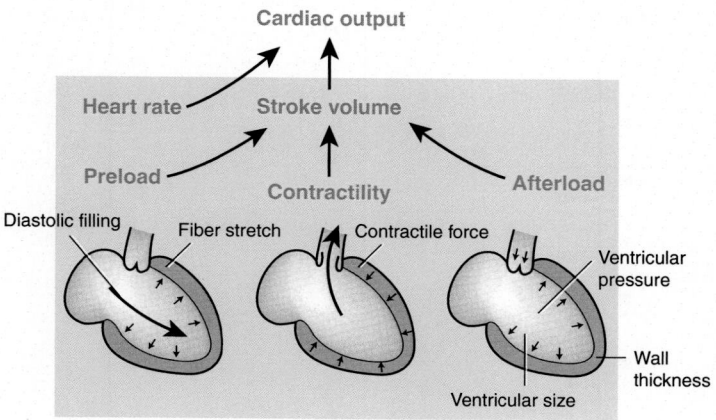

Normal CO is 4 to 8 L/min. CO may be decreased because of hypovolemia or left ventricular (LV) failure. CO may also be high (greater than 8 L/min). Even though it may seem that the higher the better, a high CO suggests hypermetabolism and associated hypoxemia usually accompanied by massive vasodilation in life-threatening conditions such as sepsis, burns, trauma, and shock.

Cardiac index (CI) is CO corrected for body size and is a more accurate parameter to monitor than CO, which varies widely depending on body surface area (BSA). Normal CI is 2.5 to 4.0 L/min/m^2.

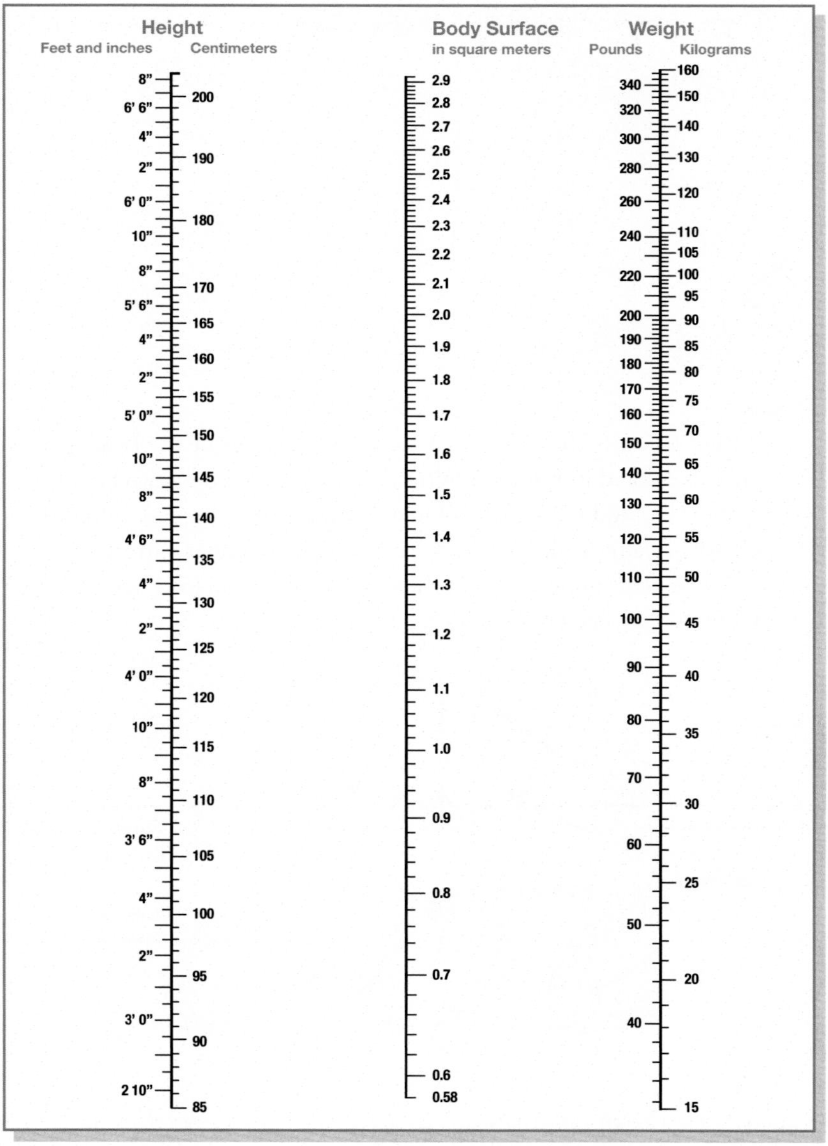

Height		Body Surface	Weight	
Feet and inches	Centimeters	in square meters	Pounds	Kilograms

Height (Feet and inches / Centimeters):
8" / 200
6' 6"
4" / 190
2"
6' 0" / 180
10"
8" / 170
5' 6" / 165
4" / 160
2" / 155
5' 0" / 150
10" / 145
8" / 140
4' 6" / 135
4" / 130
2" / 125
4' 0" / 120
10" / 115
8" / 110
3' 6" / 105
4" / 100
2" / 95
3' 0" / 90
2 10" / 85

Body Surface (in square meters):
2.9, 2.8, 2.7, 2.6, 2.5, 2.4, 2.3, 2.2, 2.1, 2.0, 1.9, 1.8, 1.7, 1.6, 1.5, 1.4, 1.3, 1.2, 1.1, 1.0, 0.9, 0.8, 0.7, 0.6, 0.58

Weight (Pounds / Kilograms):
340 / 160
320 / 150
300 / 140
280 / 130
260 / 120
240 / 110 / 105
220 / 100 / 95
200 / 90
190 / 85
180 / 80
170 / 75
160 / 70
150 / 65
140 / 60
130
120 / 55
110 / 50
100 / 45
90 / 40
80 / 35
70 / 30
60 / 25
50
40 / 20
15

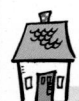

TAKE HOME POINTS

- Tracking trends in CI values is generally more useful than monitoring single data points since temporary changes may not be clinically significant.
- When the CI drops below 2.5, tissue oxygenation is compromised. The cause may be found by investigating the determinants of SV..

 $CI = \dfrac{CO}{BSA}$

BSA Nomogram

Place a straight edge so that it crosses the patient's height on the left and weight on the right. The BSA is the point at which the straight edge intersects the middle line.

A CI below 2.2 can be life-threatening.

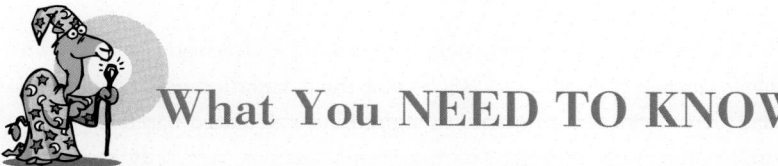

What You NEED TO KNOW

CO monitoring is indicated in clinical situations in which a concern exists regarding adequate oxygen delivery to the tissues. CO monitoring provides insight into the mechanism of the decrease in the CO so that it can be treated early and appropriately. Otherwise the problem may go unrecognized until the body's compensatory mechanisms have failed and the patient exhibits clinical signs of decreased perfusion: decreased level of consciousness; a weak, rapid, thready pulse; cool, clammy skin; and decreased urinary output.

$$CO = HR \times SV$$

Changes in the CO are influenced either by changes in HR or in the determinants of SV. HR is affected by many factors including the autonomic nervous system, metabolic rate, compensatory mechanisms, and medications. An increase in HR will increase CO up to a point. Because the ventricles fill during diastole, the faster the HR and the less time for ventricular filling. Therefore as the HR increases, eventually CO will decrease rather than increase. HR is simple to measure noninvasively.

Stroke Volume

If the CO is decreased and the HR is not the problem, then the problem lies with the SV. Each determinant of SV—preload, afterload, and contractility —must be assessed to determine the proper treatment of the patient.

Preload

The volume and the stretch of the ventricle just before systole determine preload. The hemodynamic term for LV preload is *left ventricular end–diastolic volume* (LVEDV). Because PA catheters do not measure LVEDV, pressure is used as an indicator of volume. Left ventricular end–diastolic pressure (LVEDP) is the same as the left atrial (LA) pressure (if the mitral valve is competent). The measurement of preload for the LV is obtained by wedging the PA catheter (see Chapter 7 for a thorough discussion of preload). The measurement of preload for the right ventricle (RV) is the right atrial pressure (RAP) or central venous pressure (CVP) (review Chapter 5).

Afterload

Afterload is the resistance to ventricular ejection. LV afterload is also known as *systemic vascular resistance* (SVR). SVR is the calculation used to measure afterload. Afterload is not directly measured but calculated based on other measured parameters. Afterload is important, because not only must the heart have just the right amount of fluid to pump but also it must not have to pump against extreme resistance. If it does, the heart muscle enlarges, oxygen demand is increased, and CO may decrease. A more thorough discussion of afterload is included in the SVR section.

Contractility

Contractility is the strength or vigor of the ventricular contraction. It is one of the determinants of CO along with preload and afterload. It is determined by several factors. The primary factors are changes in the stretch of the ventricular myocardium because of volume, and changes in the sympathetic activation of the ventricles. Other factors include oxygenation and electrolyte balance. Factors affecting contractility are called *inotropic agents*. Positive inotropic agents *increase* the force of contraction, and negative inotropic agents *decrease* the force of contraction.

Contractility is not directly measured. Even though a hemodynamic parameter exists called *left ventricular stroke work index* (LVSWI), it is a calculated value and not usually used clinically. SV index or stroke index (SI) is a more specific measure for individualizing SVs based on patient size. SI is used as an indirect measurement of contractility and ventricular function. Normal SI is 30 to 65 ml/beat/m^2.

$$SI = \frac{SV}{BSA}$$

In reality the SI is not assessed first. Usually the preload and afterload are assessed, and then, if a known cause of decreased CO such as heart failure exists, a positive inotropic drug is given. If contractility is thought to be too strong (i.e., in coronary artery disease where the goal is to decrease the myocardial oxygen demand), a negative inotropic drug may be prescribed.

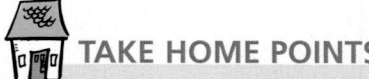

TAKE HOME POINTS

Low contractility is treated with positive inotropic drugs such as digoxin, dobutamine, milrinone, or calcium. High contractility is treated with negative inotropic agents such as beta blockers and calcium antagonists.

TAKE HOME POINTS

- Normal EF is 60% to 75%.
- EF is commonly used as the main indicator of LV function.
- EF can be determined by cardiac catheterization or echocardiogram.

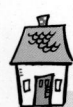

TAKE HOME POINTS

In most situations, room temperature injectate has enough of a temperature gradient to be effective. In exceptionally warm rooms such as burn units, iced injectate is recommended.

Summary

SV is defined hemodynamically as *the volume of blood in the LV at the end of diastole minus the volume at the end of systole* or *LVEDV minus left ventricular end–systolic volume* (LVESV). A simpler way to state this is the amount of blood ejected from the LV with each heartbeat. Normal SV is 60 to 130 ml, although it is not measured directly. Ejection fraction (EF) is the ratio of SV to end-diastolic volume, or the amount of blood squeezed out compared with the amount of blood remaining in the ventricle during one heartbeat. EF is expressed as a percentage. For example, if the patient has an end-diastolic volume of 100 ml and an SV of 60 ml, then his or her EF would be 60%. EF may be obtained by cardiac catheterization or noninvasively by echocardiogram.

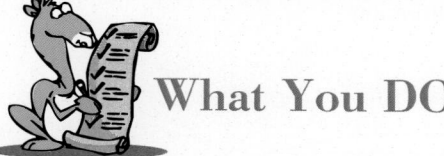

What You DO

Thermodilution Method

CO may be measured by several methods. The invasive method used most exclusively at the bedside is the thermodilution method. A specific quantity of known indicator solution with a temperature lower than that of the blood is injected into the proximal injectate port of the thermodilution PA catheter.

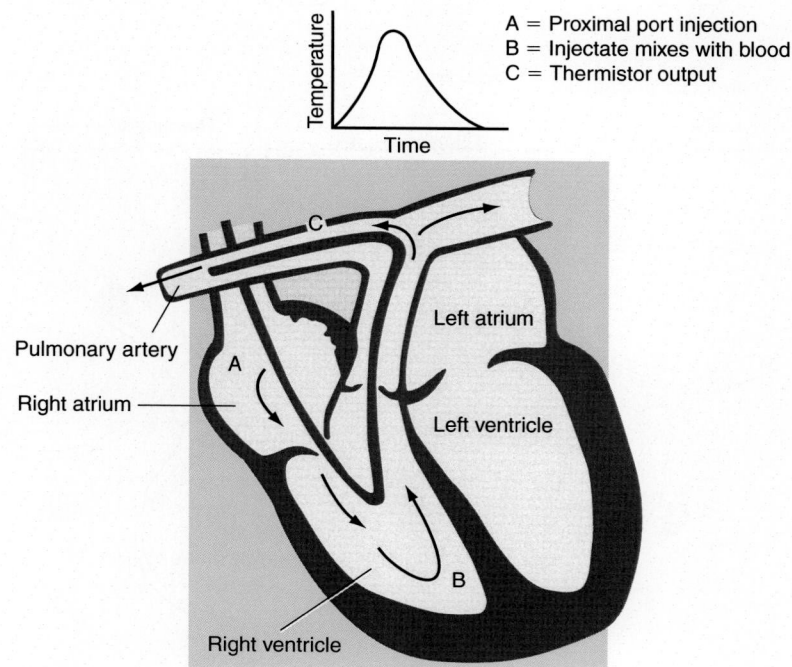

A = Proximal port injection
B = Injectate mixes with blood
C = Thermistor output

The cool injectate is introduced rapidly and smoothly as a bolus into the RA chamber. The bolus passes into the RV and is then ejected into the PA, where the temperature of the mixed blood is recorded by a thermistor at the distal end of the catheter. The monitor uses an internal formula to automatically calculate the CO from this "tagged" volume of blood.

CO may be measured continuously or intermittently. Continuous monitoring requires a special PA catheter and monitor setup. Every 30 seconds, the displayed CO is updated and reflects the average pulmonary blood flow of the previous 3 to 6 minutes. Its graphic display illustrates CO trends over time. Newer versions of the catheter display continuous CO, as well as right ventricular ejection fraction (RVEF), right ventricular end–diastolic volume (RVEDV), SV, and mixed venous saturation.

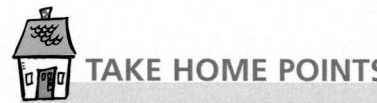

TAKE HOME POINTS

The thermistor also allows continuous monitoring of the patient's core temperature which is digitally displayed on the bedside monitor.

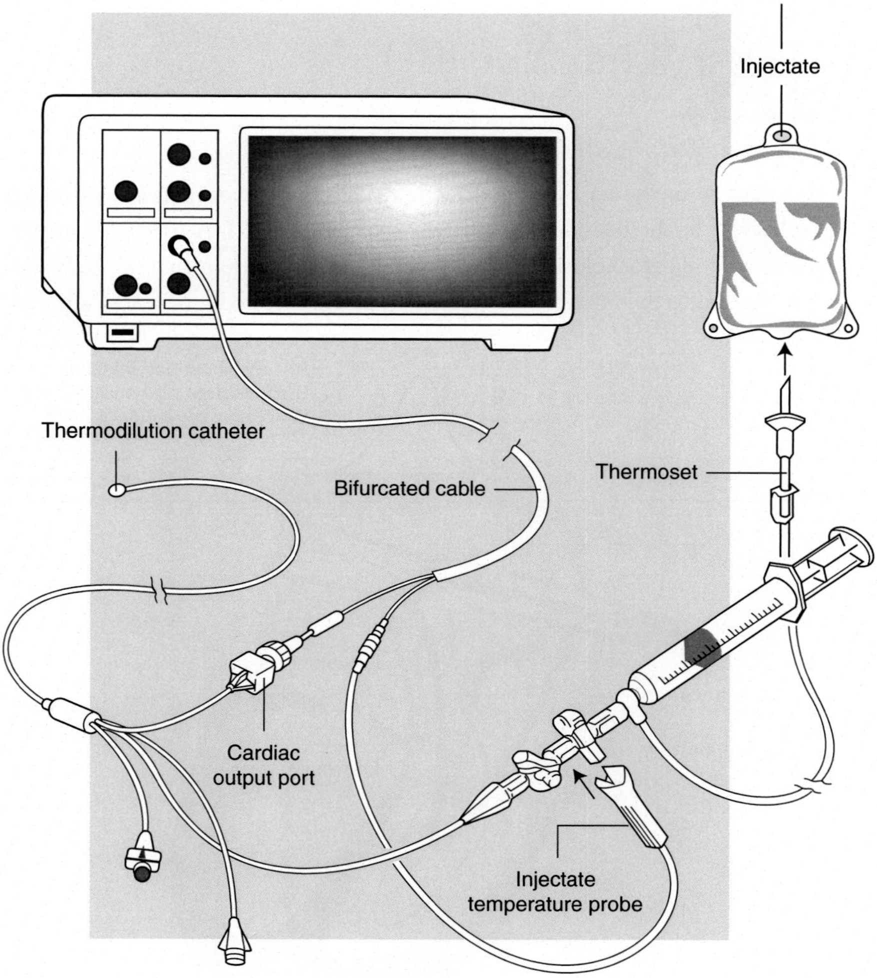

Injectate

Thermodilution catheter

Bifurcated cable

Thermoset

Cardiac output port

Injectate temperature probe

The intermittent thermodilution method is the more commonly used method. A bifurcated cable attaches the CO system to the monitor. One end is attached to the CO port on the PA catheter; the other connects to a temperature-sensing device that clips into a port on special thermoset tubing.

A thermoguard syringe keeps the solution at room temperature without warming up in the nurse's hands. A known volume of fluid at a given temperature is rapidly injected (less than 4 seconds) into the proximal injectate port of the PA catheter to enter the RA.

As this bolus of blood is ejected into the PA, a sensor near the distal tip of the PA catheter measures this change in blood temperature. CO is then computed based on the temperature change and the time it takes the injected volume to pass the thermistor. The temperature change during injection is graphically displayed on the CO computer or bedside monitor as a CO curve. The curve should be smooth with a rapid upstroke to a peak and a gradual downslope back to the baseline. Typically, three curves are obtained and the average of all three used.

The area under the curve is inversely related to the flow rate in the PA and therefore to

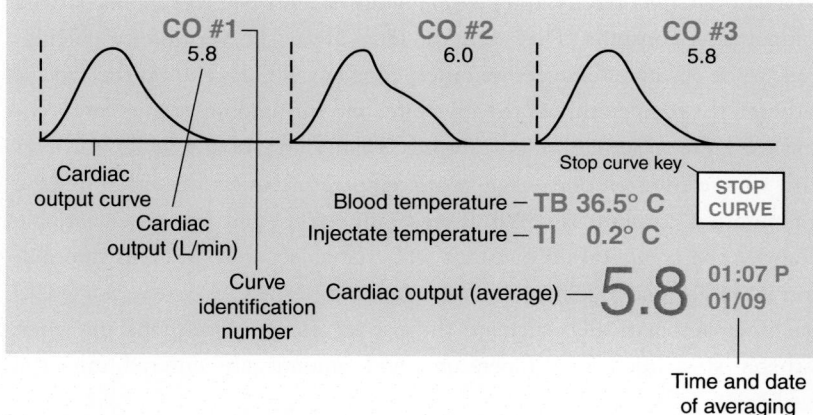

the CO. If the CO is low, the curve is low and broad and the area under the curve is large, reflecting the large temperature change in the blood that occurs from the low blood flow state. If the CO is high, the curve is tall and narrow and the area under the curve is small, indicating the lack of temperature change from the rapid movement of blood past the thermistor. An injection that is too slow may result in an irregular, faulty curve. Proper technique must be used to ensure accurate measurements.

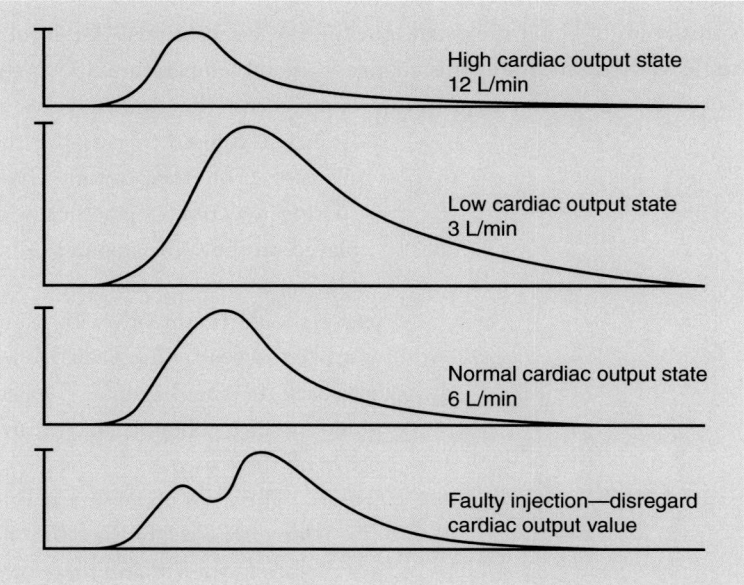

Computation Constant

To measure CO correctly, the bedside monitor must be programmed with a computation constant. This constant must always be verified for calculations to be accurate. The computation constant will depend on the type of catheter, the temperature of the injectate, and the amount of injectate solution used. For example, for an Edwards Swan-Ganz size 7.5 Fr PA catheter with venous infusion port, using room temperature injectate with 5 ml, the computation constant is 0.298. If iced saline is used or any other variable changes, the computation constant will change accordingly. This information is readily available from the manufacturer of the CO system. Some CO machines automatically calculate the correct computation constant when catheter size, injectate temperature, and amount are entered into the machine.

Cardiac Index

Most CO computers automatically do the calculation of CI if body surface information (height and weight) is available.

Troubleshooting

• The presence of valvular dysfunction or rhythm abnormalities may cause thermodilution CO values to be inaccurate.
• Technical difficulties include programming the wrong computation constant, injecting too slowly, or injecting the wrong amount or the wrong temperature solution.
• If the patient's height and weight are not entered, indexes such as CI cannot be calculated. Question marks will appear on the computation printout.

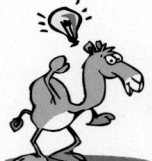

Do You UNDERSTAND?

DIRECTIONS: **Fill in the blanks to complete each of the following statements.**

1. A word that is used to describe how a drug affects the contractility of

   the heart is _____.

2. A _____ inotropic drug increases the force of contraction.

3. A _____ inotropic drug decreases the force of contraction.

4. Intermittent fluid injections for CO measurement should be injected

   _____.

5. A normal CI is _____ to _____ $L/min/m^2$.

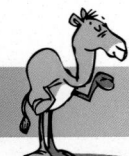

What IS Afterload?

Systemic Vascular Resistance

SVR is the major determinant in the dynamics of afterload, or the resistance the ventricles face when ejecting blood. For the purpose of this discussion, SVR will be considered synonymous with afterload. SVR is defined as *the mean resistance of all of the arterioles in the systemic circulation*. Arterioles are small branches of arteries. They have a muscular layer that can constrict or dilate in an attempt to keep the blood flowing to all of the major organs. The vascular tone of all of the arterioles in the entire body is reflected back into the aorta. The LV must pump forcefully enough to overcome the resistance that is created by this vascular tone.

Pulmonary Vascular Resistance

Pulmonary vascular resistance (PVR) is the right-sided version of SVR. It measures the resistance that the *right* ventricle must overcome rather than the left. It is a reflection of the *pulmonary* arterioles rather than the systemic. It is the afterload for the RV.

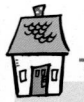

TAKE HOME POINTS

- Arterioles are resistance vessels. They have muscular walls so that they can constrict and dilate.
- SVR measures the resistance caused by arteriolar constriction or dilation.
- Venules are small veins. They are capacitance vessels. This means that they expand and collapse with volume.

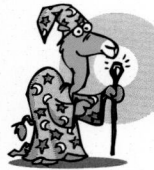

What You NEED TO KNOW

Pathophysiology

Blood pressure (BP) is determined by two factors: (1) CO and (2) SVR or afterload. BP will not reflect early clinical changes in hemodynamics because of the compensatory interaction with CO and SVR. If the CO decreases, the blood vessels will constrict in an attempt to raise the BP. This vasoconstriction causes an increase in SVR.

If something causes the blood vessels to dilate, the SVR will be decreased. If the SVR decreases, the CO will attempt to increase by increasing the rate and strength of contraction to "fill up" the larger space created by the vasodilation. These mechanisms are initially able to keep the BP within normal limits. However, over time, the CO and the BP will drop if the cause of the increased or decreased SVR is not treated. For example, if the SVR increases too much, and the heart cannot overcome the resistance, CO will fall. This leads to decreased oxygen delivery to the cells, resulting in tissue ischemia and organ dysfunction.

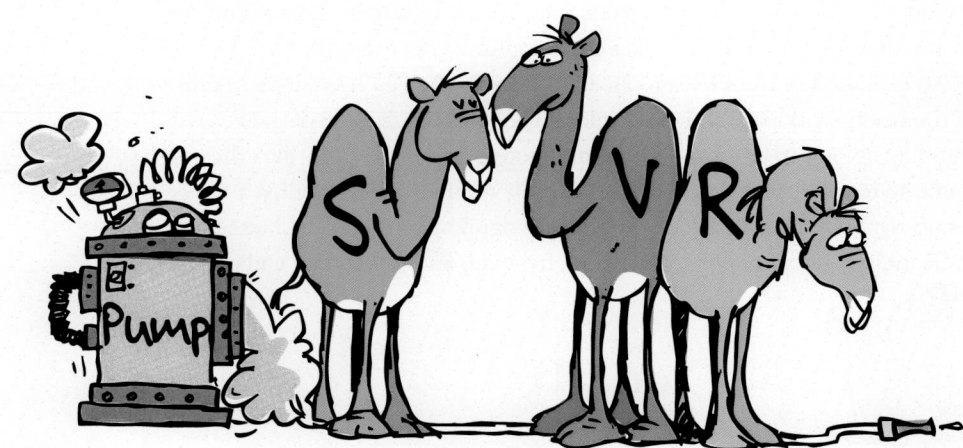

Because of these compensatory interactions, the BP is unable to signal early clinical changes in hemodynamic status. If a patient begins to bleed postoperatively, the BP will generally not reflect this change until the HR and SV increases can no longer compensate. The same situation occurs in a patient who has congestive heart failure (CHF) or a myocardial infarction (MI). BP will not reflect the early changes in hemodynamics, because compensatory mechanisms serve to keep the BP normal.

Systemic Vascular Resistance and Pulmonary Vascular Resistance Measurement

SVR and PVR should be calculated whenever a PA catheter is available. SVR is especially useful in hypotension of unknown cause and to help judge the effectiveness of drug intervention. BP can fall as the result of increased or decreased peripheral resistance.

SVR monitoring can help differentiate whether the blood vessels are constricted or dilated; therefore it can be used to determine the appropriate treatment. For example, in cardiogenic shock, the blood vessels will constrict in an attempt to keep the blood circulating. This patient needs positive inotropic support (a drug to help the heart pump more forcefully) and a vasodilator to decrease resistance to that pumping. However, in septic shock, which may produce the same BP clinically, the SVR will be decreased because the blood vessels are dilated. The CO will be elevated. This patient needs a lot of intravenous (IV) fluid to fill up this expanded space and a vasopressor to "tighten up" the space.

If the SVR is elevated, the LV will face an increased resistance to the ejection of blood. In an acute setting such as shock, this is a desired response. However, a chronic increase in SVR causes systemic hypertension.

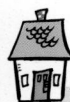

Medications affecting afterload exert their effects by either vasoconstricting or vasodilating the muscular layer of the walls of the arterioles.

An elevation of the PVR produces a strain on the RV. It enlarges because of the heavy workload, and over time the RV will fail. Failure of the RV will cause less blood to enter the lungs and more blood to back up into the systemic system. This increased workload can eventually affect the LV, and systemic hypotension can occur. The most common causes of an increase in PVR include pulmonary hypertension, hypoxia, and pulmonary emboli.

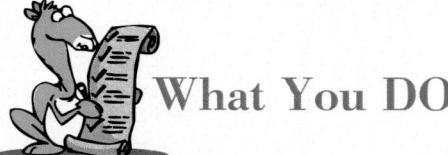

What You DO

Calculations

No waveform exists for SVR because it is not a directly measured parameter. It is derived from values obtained from the PA catheter and is calculated by the following formula:

$$SVR = \frac{MAP - RAP \times 80}{CO}$$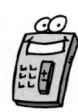

The resulting measurement is not in mm Hg but in dynes/sec/cm^{-5}. This is a resistance measurement. The following formula is for PVR:

$$PVR = \frac{mean\ PA\ pressure - PAOP \times 80}{CO}$$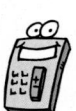

Treatment

Several options exist for treating a high SVR:
- IV sodium nitroprusside is used in the acute setting to rapidly decrease SVR, as in a patient with the back pain of an aortic aneurysm and malignant hypertension.
- Fenoldopam is a newer drug that also has been shown to decrease SVR in severe hypertension.
- In the less acute setting, angiotensin-converting enzyme (ACE) inhibitors indirectly vasodilate and therefore serve as afterload reducers.
- The mechanics of the intraaortic balloon pump also affect SVR. The balloon pump inflates during diastole to enhance coronary blood supply. It deflates during systole to decrease afterload.

If the SVR is low, the LV faces a lower resistance to the ejection of blood. A "relative hypovolemia" exists, because the blood vessels dilate and inadequate volume exists to fill up the space. The nurse should:

- Give fluid boluses to sustain an adequate BP.
- If ordered, administer vasopressor drugs such as epinephrine, norepinephrine, Neo-Synephrine, and dopamine at high levels to increase SVR in cases of massive vasodilation. Clinical examples include anaphylaxis and septic shock. If the underlying condition is not treated, the use of vasopressors will provide only short-term success.

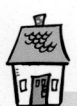

TAKE HOME POINTS

- Fluid boluses and vasopressor drugs are used to treat a low SVR.
- Vasodilators are used to treat a high SVR.

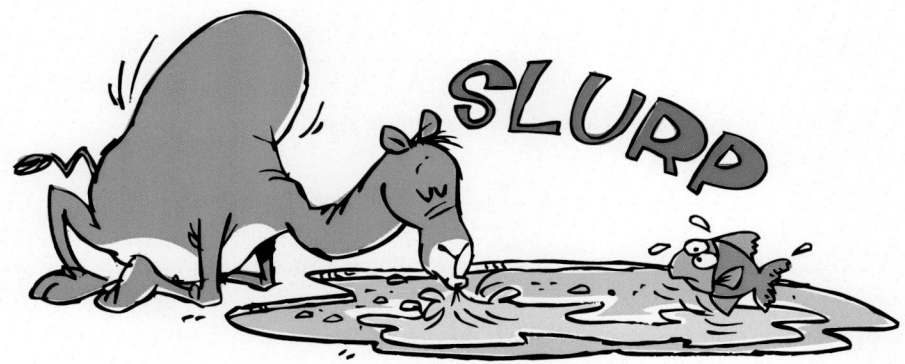

Troubleshooting

Because the measurements of SVR and PVR are essentially obtained by calculation method rather than direct measurement, it is most important to ensure that the parameters used for calculation (MAP, CVP, CO) are accurate.

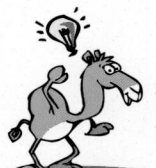

Do You UNDERSTAND?

DIRECTIONS: **Match each statement in Column A with an answer in Column B.**

Column A	Column B
_____ 1. Afterload for the systemic circulation	a. SVR
_____ 2. Afterload for the pulmonary circulation	b. PVR

DIRECTIONS: **Fill in the blanks to complete each of the following statements.**

3. A patient in hypovolemic shock would have a(n)_____ in SVR. The main treatment needed in this patient is

_____   _____

_____.

4. Vasodilators are used to help _____ SVR.

5. When the intraaortic balloon deflates during systole, it decreases

_____.

DIRECTIONS: **Provide an answer to the following questions.**

6. The main determinant of SVR is the constriction and dilation of what type of vessels?

_____

7. MAP is determined by the interrelationship of which two variables?

_____

_____

8. Hemodynamic parameters including an elevated CO and a low SVR

are classic signs of _____   _____.

Mixed Venous Oxygenation Monitoring

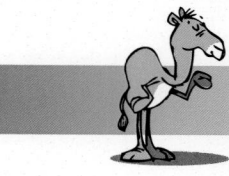

What IS Mixed Venous Oxygen Saturation Monitoring?

Mixed venous oxygen saturation (SvO_2) is the measure of the amount of oxygen in the hemoglobin (Hb) in venous blood that has returned to the right ventricle (RV) and the pulmonary artery (PA). SvO_2 monitoring allows the study of the balance between oxygen supply and demand in the body. It is determined by the tissue oxygen consumption and the amount of blood pumped out of the heart (cardiac output).

Changes in SvO_2 will long precede changes in cardiac output and other monitoring information that are available to the bedside nurse. By monitoring SvO_2, it gives the nurse a jump on detecting and preventing changes that may have adverse effects on patients.

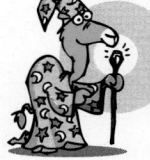

What You NEED TO KNOW

Blood is designed to carry both oxygen and carbon dioxide. Hb, a molecule inside the blood, has four binding sites that oxygen molecules can occupy. The more oxygen that is breathed in, the more oxygen will stick to Hb's binding sites (saturation). When Hb is 100% saturated, no more oxygen can be transported on it. The amount of oxygen stuck to these Hb binding sites corresponds to a partial pressure of oxygen in the blood.

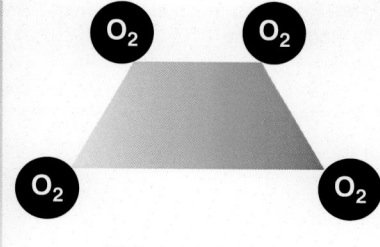

Although oxygen binds to Hb, it does not stay bound indefinitely. If it did, the oxygen would never move off the Hb and into the cells and cells would die. Instead, oxygen molecules release themselves from the Hb and move (diffuse) to areas (cells) with less oxygen molecules. This exchange of oxygen from Hb to the cells continues until equilibrium is reached.

On breathing in (inspiration), oxygen attaches to Hb and creates partial pressure of oxygen (PaO_2) in the arterial blood. The relationship between PaO_2 and how well saturated with oxygen Hb is, is called *arterial oxygen saturation* (SaO_2).

It is a myth that arterial blood is oxygenated and venous blood is deoxygenated. Even after the cells take the oxygen they need, some oxygen is still left in the venous blood supply. A sample of venous blood from a healthy, normal human would still have an oxygen saturation of about 75%. The human body, under normal conditions, makes far more oxygen available to the cells than the cells can use.

Mixed SvO_2 is the result of many factors:

$$SvO_2 = SaO_2 - (\text{oxygen consumed} \times \text{Hb} \times \text{cardiac output})$$

Low SvO_2 has two main categorical causes:
1. A decrease in oxygen supply to the tissues
2. An increase in oxygen use because of a high demand

If the amount of Hb in the blood is low, then oxygen delivery will also be low because fewer molecules are available to carry oxygen to the tissues. Blood loss can result in a decreased supply of oxygen to the tissues and a decreased SvO_2 level.

A decrease in oxygen supply can also result from low cardiac output. Causes of an increase in oxygen demand include pain, stress, shivering and hyperthermia, and seizures. The SvO_2 level will drop as the supply of oxygen falls below the oxygen demand of the body. Simple procedures such as turning, bathing, and suctioning will also cause a decrease in SvO_2 as a result of increased oxygen demand from activity.

TAKE HOME POINTS

- Oxygen is in the bloodstream only so it can be carried to the cells of the body, where it provides power for the cells to do their work.

- In a normal, healthy adult, only about 25% of the oxygen taken into the body is used.

- It is important to remember that Hb count and SaO_2 are **NOT** the same. SaO_2 is the amount of oxygen sticking to the Hb binding sites. Hb counts are directly related to blood volume.

An SvO_2 below 60%
indicates that oxygen
supply is too low or
the oxygen demand is too
high. A low oxygen supply
and an SvO_2 below 60% is
indicative of heart failure and
an SvO_2 reading below 40%
indicates profound shock. A
demand for too much oxygen
and an SvO_2 below 60% is
indicative of hypothyroidism
or sepsis. At an SvO_2 level
below 30%, anaerobic
metabolism (metabolism
without oxygen) occurs and
lactic acidosis begins to
develop in the tissues.

CAUSES OF CHANGES IN MIXED VENOUS OXYGEN SATURATION

Low SvO_2

Increased Oxygen Demand

Increased metabolic rate	Hyperthermia
Seizures	Shivering
Pain	Anxiety
Stress	Strenuous exercise

In a compromised patient, normal activities can also increase oxygen demand

Decreased Oxygen Supply

Anemia	
Hemorrhage	
Ventilation-perfusion mismatches	Lung disease
Low cardiac output	Hypovolemia
Heart failure	Shock
Myocardial infarction	

High SvO_2

Decreased Oxygen Demand

Sepsis (early stages)	Hypothermia
Anesthesia	

Increased Oxygen Supply

Supplemental oxygen
Other causes:
  Wedged pulmonary artery catheter
  Clot at tip of catheter

TAKE HOME POINTS

A SvO_2 level greater than 80% indicates either a technical error, that the oxygen supply is too high (need to turn down the amount of inspired oxygen [FIO_2]), or that the oxygen demand is low. A low oxygen demand with an SvO_2 greater than 80% is indicative of hypothermia, anesthesia, hypothyroidism, and early sepsis.

Certain disease states cause the SvO_2 to be high or appear normal despite inadequate tissue oxygenation. Basically the SvO_2 reading is high because the tissues are unable to extract the regular amount of oxygen. This results in more oxygen returning back to the pulmonary arteries where SvO_2 is measured.

Sepsis (an infection), is a situation that would result in an increased SvO_2 reading despite a lack of oxygen to the tissues. Other causes include any condition resulting in shunting of blood between the arterial and venous systems. A shunt means that blood flows from an artery to a vein without losing its carbon dioxide in the lung.

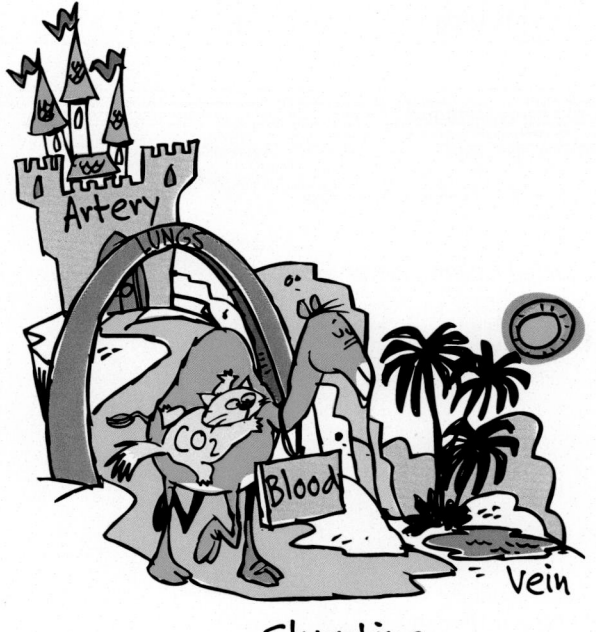

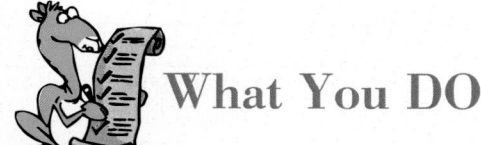

Arteriovenous shunts and intracardiac shunts, connections between the ventricles or atria of the heart through the septum, will result in oxygenated blood bypassing the tissues and returning to the venous system back to the PA where SvO_2 is measured. Other causes include cirrhosis of the liver, cyanide poisoning, and unintentional PA catheter wedging.

What You DO

To measure the oxygen consumption and extraction, the physician needs to measure venous samples of blood from the PA through a PA catheter.

Inserting a mixed venous oxygen catheter only requires a couple more steps than inserting a PA catheter. (Review the nurse's responsibilities and the procedure for PA catheter insertion in Chapter 6.)

The PA catheter used to measure SvO_2 is inserted into a large vein such as the jugular vein or, more infrequently, the subclavian vein. The catheter is passed through a device called an *introducer* that has been placed into the vein. To determine where to place the catheter tip, a waveform and pressure monitor are used to guide the catheter into position. The PA catheter is

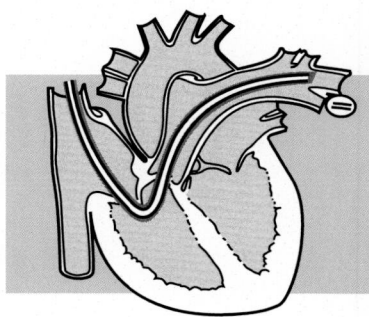

Pulmonary artery wedge pressure

Normal range
Mean: 4-12 mm Hg

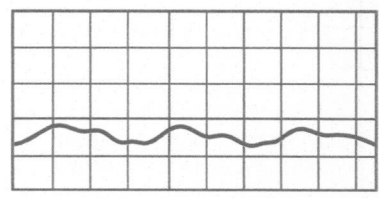

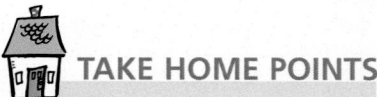

TAKE HOME POINTS

Strict sterile technique must be maintained throughout the insertion of the catheter.

threaded through the introducer, into position through the vena cava, and into the right atrium (RA). Once the catheter tip is in the RA, the balloon on the pulmonary catheter is inflated with air. This helps the catheter "float" through the tricuspid valve and into the RV. The balloon then floats across the pulmonic valve into the PA and finally into the wedged position.

The nurse assisting the physician should monitor the patient's electrocardiogram (ECG) during catheter insertion for any kind of abnormal beating of the heart (ectopy). As the tip of the catheter passes through the RV, the direct stimulation of the catheter on this part of the heart may cause abnormal beats to occur.

The only additional step for the insertion of an SvO_2 PA catheter is to take a sample of blood from the mixed venous oxygen port (distal port) to measure the amount of oxygen in the sample. Once the reading is complete, the mixed venous oxygen computer is calibrated. The device is then set to monitor continuously by hooking a cable connection to the PA catheter. Automatic updates give a continuous mixed venous oxygen consumption reading. The nurse should chart these readings at the intervals ordered and be alert for readings that show the patient might be headed for trouble.

Treating a low SvO_2 includes increasing the oxygen supply by means of supplemental oxygen, blood transfusions, drugs, and fluid management to increase cardiac output, and identifying and eliminating the cause if the low reading has resulted from a high demand.

If the patient increases the amount of oxygen he or she consumes, then the mixed SvO_2 decreases. This can happen if someone has a disease that increases his or her work of breathing. The tissues are consuming more of the oxygen supply, with less being left in the blood where it can be measured. To increase the mixed SvO_2, the nurse should:

- Add more oxygen, using a nasal cannula or more advanced devices.
- Cut back on the patient's oxygen consumption by administering drugs, if ordered, that ease the work of breathing. Judicious use of sedative and analgesics can help ease the work of breathing and are often used before the use of neuromuscular blockade. In addition, nondepolarizing neuromuscular blockers also can be used; however, neuromuscular blockers require endotracheal intubation and mechanical ventilation. Bronchodilators may work if the patient has a large airway obstruction or spasm, but SvO_2 is not ordinarily acutely affected by such a change.

If the patient increases oxygen consumption, then the arterial oxygen saturation (SaO_2) begins to decrease and the SvO_2 begins to drop. To increase mixed SvO_2, the nurse should add more oxygen, using a nasal cannula or more advanced devices.

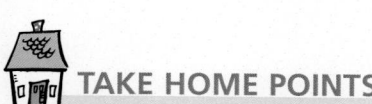

TAKE HOME POINTS

It is not necessary to have an SvO_2 PA catheter to draw an SvO_2 sample. These can be drawn from the PA distal port of any PA catheter. An SvO_2 catheter is needed for continuous SvO_2 monitoring.

Giving the nondepolarizing neuromuscular–blocking drugs without ventilating the patient will cause death.

In patients with decreased Hb counts because of bleeding, SvO_2 drops. The Hb count can be corrected by the administration of blood. (Follow institutional protocols and procedures for blood administration.)

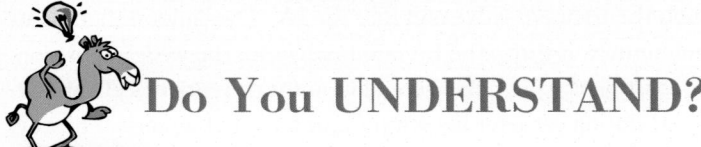

Do You UNDERSTAND?

DIRECTIONS: **Fill in the blanks to complete each of the following statements.**

1. When oxygen molecules leave the blood and reenter the blood at the

   same rate, _____ has been achieved.

2. If SaO_2 is 100% and mixed SvO_2 is 60%, then the body is using

   _____%.

3. Name four things that can cause mixed venous saturation levels to drop.

   _____

   _____

   _____

   _____

4. An SvO_2 of 40% indicates _____

   _____.

DIRECTIONS: On the following graph, use the oxyhemoglobin dissociation curve to identify the partial pressure of oxygen and the oxygen saturation at various points, indicated by letters. (*Sample: 96 mm Hg partial pressure, 96% saturation.*)

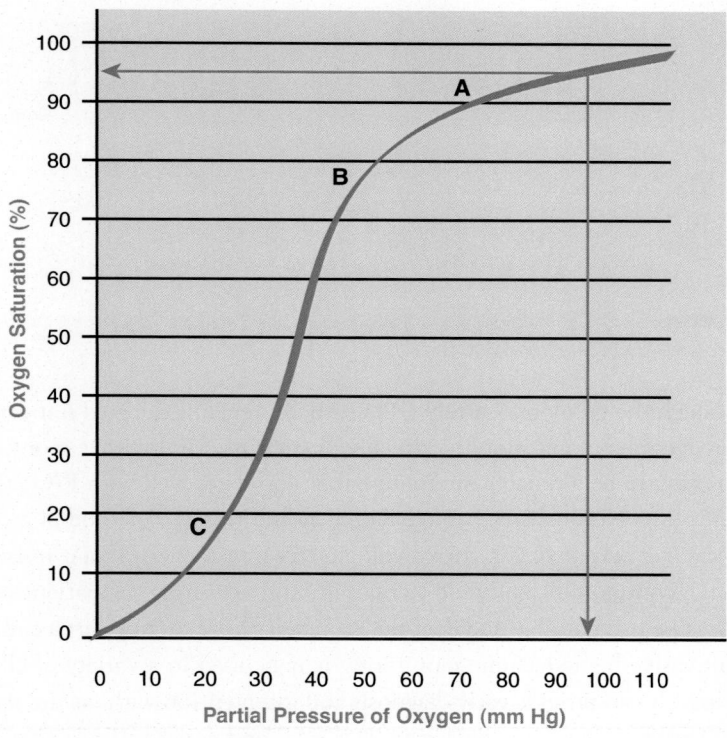

A. _____ partial pressure, _____ saturation

B. _____ partial pressure, _____ saturation

C. _____ partial pressure, _____ saturation

10 Noninvasive Hemodynamic Monitoring

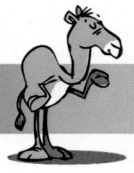

What IS Noninvasive Hemodynamic Monitoring?

Although the pulmonary artery (PA) catheter remains the gold standard for hemodynamic monitoring in critically ill patients, noninvasive monitoring is proving to be a reliable alternative that correlates well with PA catheter monitoring. Noninvasive hemodynamic monitoring is a method of measuring cardiac output (CO), stroke volume (SV), systemic vascular resistance (SVR), contractility, and fluid status without puncturing the patient's skin.

Because it is portable and does not require a physician to insert a catheter, noninvasive hemodynamic monitoring may be used in a variety of clinical settings. It can provide early diagnosis and intervention without the risks of conventional invasive monitoring. It is safer and easier to learn than conventional hemodynamic monitoring. Current systems are user friendly, easy to apply, and reproducible. Results can be obtained in less than 5 minutes after proper connection to equipment.

With noninvasive hemodynamic monitoring, data are obtained in a different manner from conventional invasive monitoring. Computer algorithms are used to measure pulsatile changes (impedance) in the electrical conductivity of the thorax (thoracic electrical bioimpedance [TEB]). The pulsatile changes are analyzed to determine SV, CO, indices of myocardial contractility, and afterload. The application of TEB technology for measuring cardiac hemodynamic function is termed *impedance cardiography* (ICG).

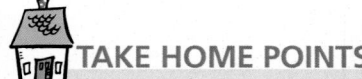

TAKE HOME POINTS

Esophageal Doppler monitoring (EDM) is a form of hemodynamic monitoring which is considered noninvasive by strict definition but is actually minimally invasive as it involves advancing a pencil-thin ultrasound probe through the patient's esophagus to a location posterior to the heart. For more information on EDM, see the Appendix A.

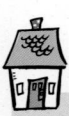

TAKE HOME POINTS

Advantages of ICG:

- Less invasive—no risk of complications
- Earlier diagnosis—results in 5 minutes—minimal set-up
- Portable—many clinical applications
- Accurate—comparable to PA catheter in most situations

Disadvantages of ICG:

- Cost—reimbursement questionable until more broadly accepted
- Learning curve—entirely new standard of measurement
- Accuracy variable in certain patients—sepsis, severe arrhythmias

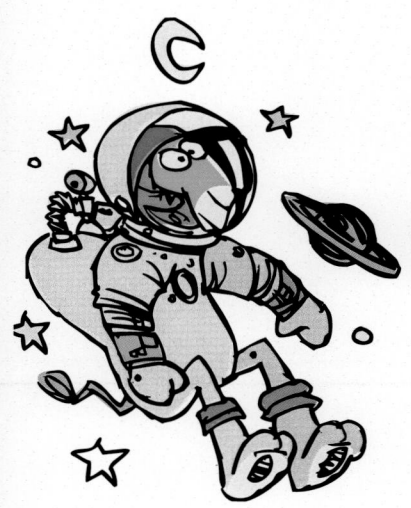

ICG provides clinical assessment that can help guide medical therapy, determine therapeutic interventions, and assist in determining prognoses. One of the more common clinical applications thus far is in the medical management of heart failure. As in all monitoring techniques, serial trending with careful correlation with the patient's clinical and laboratory profile is essential to forming sound diagnostic and therapeutic judgments. As technology becomes more advanced and more validation studies are reported, it is possible that noninvasive monitoring may eventually replace invasive hemodynamic monitoring.

ICG is an exciting new application of an older technology. The concept of monitoring hemodynamics through skin electrodes was originally used by the National Aeronautics and Space Administration (NASA) in the 1960s. It was used to evaluate the effects of zero gravity on astronauts. Although at the time it worked well in healthy adults, it was not considered accurate in critically ill patients. Since the advent of the microprocessor, technologic advances in echocardiography and magnetic resonance imaging (MRI), and a better understanding of the cardiac cycle, ICG is now considered as reliable and accurate as a PA catheter in most cases.

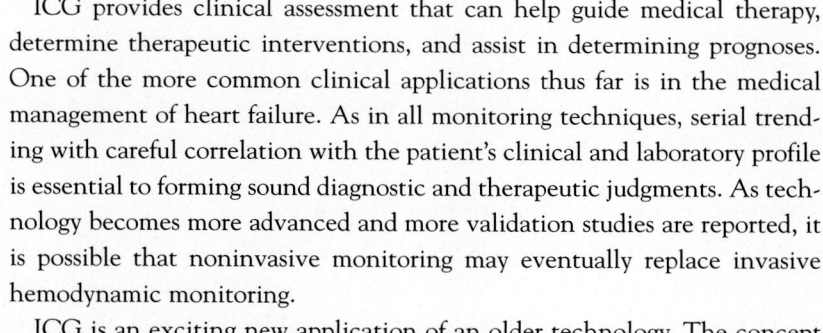

What You NEED TO KNOW

How Impedance Cardiography Works

The amount of electrical energy that can flow through any substance relates to the size and the inherent conductivity of that substance. Certain substances are good conductors of electrical energy, whereas other substances resist (impede) the flow of energy. For example, air and bone are poor conductors (high impedance), whereas fluid such as blood in the heart and great vessels of the thorax is a good conductor (low impedance). To measure the electrical conductivity of an object and its impedance, electrical energy of a known, constant voltage is introduced into that object. The amount of voltage is measured at a location that is removed from the area where it was introduced. The difference in the amount of voltage between what was introduced and was measured is an indicator of the impedance to the flow of energy through that object. If the object is the thorax, changes in impedance

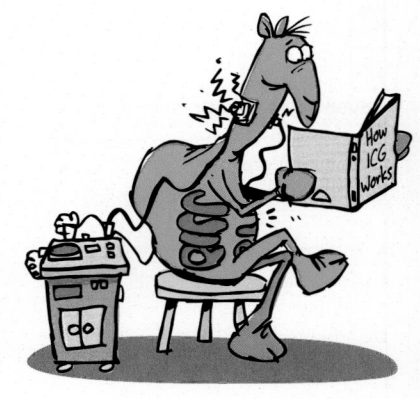

over time can be recorded in numeric values and graphed as a waveform similar to an electrocardiogram (ECG) waveform and correlated with the ECG.

ICG works by converting changes in TEB into changes in volume over time in relation to the cardiac cycle. In this manner, it is used to track volumetric changes such as those occurring during the cardiac cycle.

How Impedance Cardiography is Measured

Four pairs of specialized, self-adhesive sensor electrodes are placed on the patient, one pair on either side of the base of the neck and one pair on either side of the lower thorax. The pads are connected by cable to a computer module.

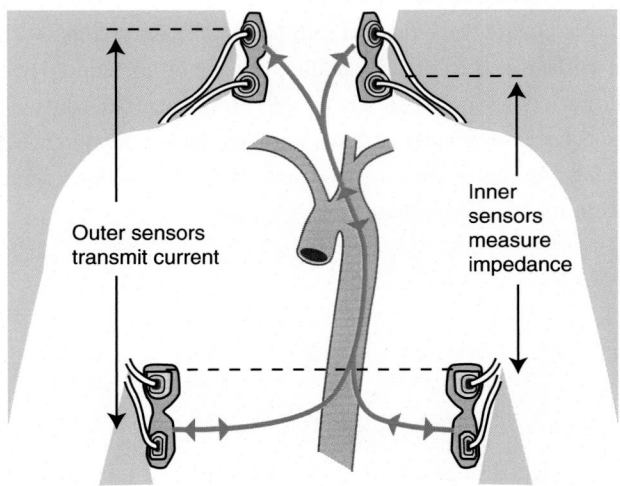

Outer sensors transmit current

Inner sensors measure impedance

A harmless, low-voltage, high-amplitude current is introduced through the outer set of electrodes placed on the neck and the lower thorax. The conducted voltage is sensed through an inner set of electrodes placed at the base of the neck and the thorax on top of the first set. The drop in voltage (or difference between what is introduced and what is sensed) is used to determine impedance (resistance) to the current.

With each heartbeat, changes in conductivity occur as blood distends, and then leaves the aorta. This pulsatile flow generates electrical impedance changes that can be recorded as a "change in impedance over changes in time" waveform. The impedance waveform is similar to an arterial pressure waveform but based on volume and velocity of aortic blood flow rather than pressure.

Q = Start of ventricular
     depolarization

B = Opening of pulmonic
     and aortic valves

C = Maximal deflection

X = Closure of aortic valve

Y = Closure of pulmonic valve

O = Mitral opening snap and
     rapid filling of ventricles

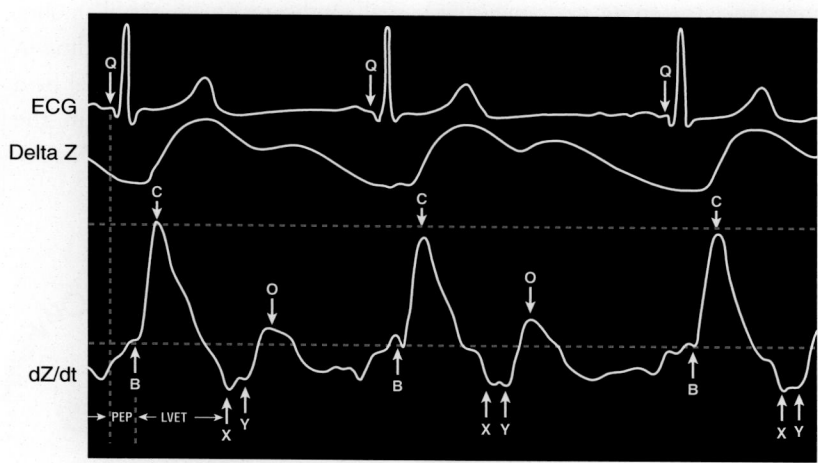

Preejection period (PEP) is measured from Q to B.
Left ventricular ejection time (LVET) is measured from B to X.

The ECG is recorded and the timing of changes in impedance is simultaneously measured and recorded. The patient's blood pressure data is entered into the computer. Algorithms are used to calculate or derive heart rate (HR), SV, CO, indices of contractility, and indices of workload. These are displayed on a monitor screen.

Impedance waveform   **Ascending aorta tracing**   **ECG waveform**

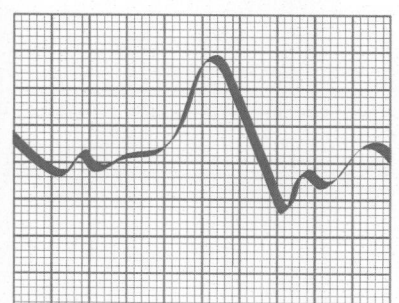 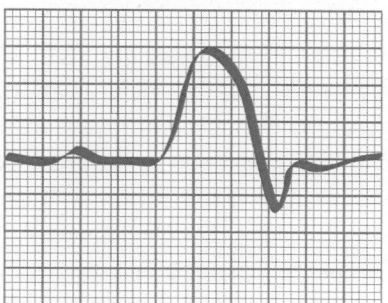 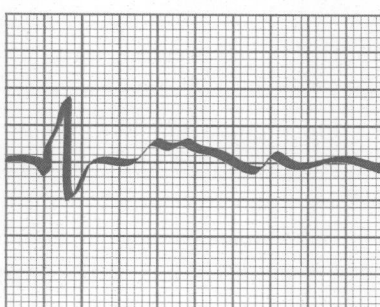

How Impedance Cardiography Detects Problems

If a change in impedance occurs, over changes in time, while the current is held constant, there must be a change in the properties of the conducting medium. It is important to remember that blood and plasma are excellent conductors of electricity. Air, bone, and other tissues, on the other hand, are not. Because intravascular volume in the chest is relatively constant, low impedance (meaning *good conduction*) usually indicates an abnormal amount of fluid in the chest from conditions such as pulmonary edema, bleeding in the thoracic cavity, or pleural effusions. In ICG, preload is measured by a parameter called *thoracic fluid content*. Greater amounts of fluid in the intravascular, interstitial, or intracellular spaces reduce TEB. The average or baseline thoracic impedance for thoracic fluid content should be between 20 and 30 ohms. If it is less than 20 ohms, then extra fluid in the chest usually exists. An increase in impedance is the goal of most interventions. The dynamics of ventilation contribute very little to any overall impedance changes.

A rapid drop in impedance can point to intrathoracic bleeding in the fresh, postoperative heart surgery patient, whereas a gradual decrease in impedance is typical of pulmonary edema. If both impedance and CO are low, the fluid accumulation is probably heart failure rather than a pulmonary problem.

Volume-depleted states such as dehydration, emphysema, and pneumothorax can increase impedance.

TAKE HOME POINTS

This is how ICG works:

- an alternating current is transmitted through the chest
- the current seeks the path of least resistance—the blood-filled aorta
- baseline impedance to current is measured
- blood volume and velocity in the aorta change with each heartbeat
- corresponding changes in impedance are used with the ECG to provide hemodynamic parameters

Indications

ICG may be used in a variety of clinical settings. It is well suited to the hospital bedside, physician's office, emergency department (ED), intensive care unit (ICU), and operating room (OR) settings. It can be used in the critical care setting to assess baseline hemodynamic status, trend changes, and monitor drug titration and fluid management, especially in patients where invasive procedures would be contraindicated. ICG would also be the preferred method of monitoring in patients who are at high risk of infection. It can help differentiate cardiogenic from pulmonary causes of acute dyspnea.

ICG may also be used in the surgery or anesthesia setting to assess hemodynamic status especially during thoracic or vascular surgery in high-risk patients. It is especially appropriate for cardiac surgery patients who are "fast tracked" to telemetry units 8 to 12 hours postoperatively. The device may be used in the ED to guide a differential diagnosis or establish baseline status on any patient with potentially unstable hemodynamics. This would include patients with heart failure, chronic obstructive pulmonary disease (COPD), hypotension, hypertension, myocardial infarction (MI), cardiac arrhythmia, trauma, and early sepsis or shock. It can be used to assess the hemodynamic status of patients on medical floors, often eliminating the

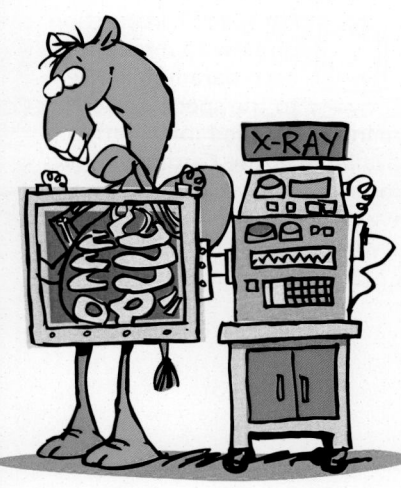

need for an invasive catheter and the need for transfer to an ICU bed. It can be used in a clinic or office setting to follow-up patients with heart failure, chest pain, hypertension, or renal failure. It can also help optimize pacemaker settings on an outpatient basis.

Research has shown that low-impedance readings are closely related to abnormal chest x-rays in heart failure patients. Detection of low CO states in heart failure patients can dramatically improve their treatment regimen. Studies also report the effectiveness of ICG as a marker for coronary artery disease during stress testing, as an early warning system for acute heart transplant rejection, and as a way to detect hemodynamic trends during laparoscopic surgery. The CO component, when combined with respiratory monitoring, has been shown to make a prognostic difference in determining which trauma victims were most likely to survive.

Contraindications

ICG may not be accurate in patients with valvular disease, left-to-right shunts, or severe pulmonary edema. Some studies have shown that the CO component does not correlate as well in critically ill patients and in patients with tachycardia, low CO, and dysrhythmias. Absolute contraindications include patients with impedance-driven pacemakers that calculate minute ventilation to regulate pulse generator pacing rate. The ICG current can interfere with the pacemaker current and may cause pacemaker rate acceleration. Other contraindications include:

- Patients with severe septic shock
- Patients who weigh less than 67 or greater than 341 pounds
- Patients whose height is less than 4 feet or greater than 7 feet 5 inches
- Patients with a HR less than 40 beats per minute (bpm) or greater than 250 bpm

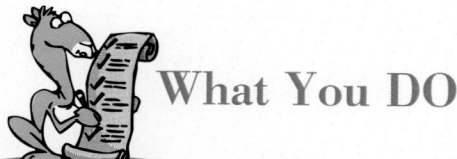

What You DO

Impedance Cardiography Equipment Setup

Equipment manufacturers offer training specific to their types of monitoring systems. It is important to become familiar with the specific operator's manual for proper placement of electrodes, patient positioning, and calibration of the machine. Operation of equipment and troubleshooting guidelines should be included in this training. The nurse's role includes recording, interpreting, and relaying findings to the physician.

Impedance Cardiography Measurement Interpretation

Because ICG uses resistance measures rather than intravascular pressures, a different standard of measurement exists that requires an entirely different focus of interpretation. Resistance is measured in ohms.

For specific instruction on how to measure each parameter, refer to the specific operator manual. Detailed information is available at the Cardiodynamics International web site at www.cardiodynamics.com or www.impedancecardiography.com.

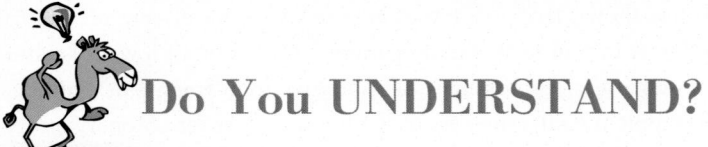

Do You UNDERSTAND?

DIRECTIONS: **Fill in the blanks to complete each of the following statements.**

1. A form of noninvasive hemodynamic monitoring using impedance as a

   measure is called _____.

2. To detect cardiac impedance, four pairs of electrodes are used; two pairs

   are placed on the chest and two on the _____.

3. An increased amount of fluid in the chest can be detected by

   _____ impedance.

4. ICG is measured in _____.

5. An absolute contraindication to the use of ICG is

   _____.

11 Clinical Applications

This chapter includes tables, exercises, and case studies to help integrate information presented in the other chapters. The following table summarizes how hemodynamic parameters assist in differential diagnoses.

How Hemodynamic Parameters Assist in Differential Diagnoses

CONDITION	DESCRIPTION	CHARACTERISTIC HEMODYNAMIC FINDINGS	
Hypovolemia	May be the result of massive blood loss, burns, third spacing, dehydration	Decreased BP Decreased CVP Increased SVR	Decreased CO Decreased PA pressures Decreased PAOP
Pulmonary edema	Caused by heart failure	Increased BP, then decreased BP Increased CVP Increased PA pressures Increased PAOP Increased SVR	Decreased CO
Adult respiratory distress syndrome	Noncardiac pulmonary edema	Increased BP, then decreased BP Increased CVP Increased PA pressures Normal-slightly increased PAOP	Increased CO
Cardiogenic shock	Failure of the heart to pump adequately	Increased CVP Increased PA pressures Increased PAOP Increased SVR	Decreased CO Decreased BP

How Hemodynamic Parameters Assist in Differential Diagnoses—cont'd

CONDITION	DESCRIPTION	CHARACTERISTIC HEMODYNAMIC FINDINGS	
Pulmonary hypertension	Common in COPD patients; could be from pulmonary embolus; no heart involvement	Increased PA pressures	Variable PAOP
Sepsis and septic shock	Dilated capillaries as the result of infectious process	Increased CO	Decreased BP Decreased PA pressures Decreased CVP Decreased PAOP or plus or minus Decreased SVR
Mitral regurgitation	Reflux into the LA during ventricular systole	Increased PAOP	
Constrictive pericarditis	Scarring of pericardium interferes withfilling, especially in right heart	Increased PAOP Increased CVP Increased PAP	Decreased CO

BP, Blood pressure; *CO,* cardiac output; *CVP,* central venous pressure; *PA,* pulmonary artery; *SVR,* systemic vascular resistance; *PAOP,* pulmonary artery occlusion pressure; *COPD,* chronic obstructive pulmonary disease; *LA,* left atrium.

- If the pulmonary artery occlusion pressure (PAOP) is low at the same time the cardiac output (CO) (stroke volume [SV]) is low, hypovolemia is assumed.
- If the PAWP/PAOP is high (usually greater than 18 mm Hg) at the same time the CO (SV) is low, left ventricular (LV) dysfunction is assumed.
- When the PAWP/PAOP and the CO (SV) are normal, then normovolemia and acceptable LV function are assumed.
- If the systemic vascular resistance (SVR) is low and the CO is high, suspect septic shock.
- If the PAWP/PAOP is normal but the pulmonary artery diastolic (PAD) is elevated, the problem is either a pulmonary embolus, pulmonary hypertension, mitral regurgitation, or mitral stenosis.

Exercise 1

Identify the following waveforms.

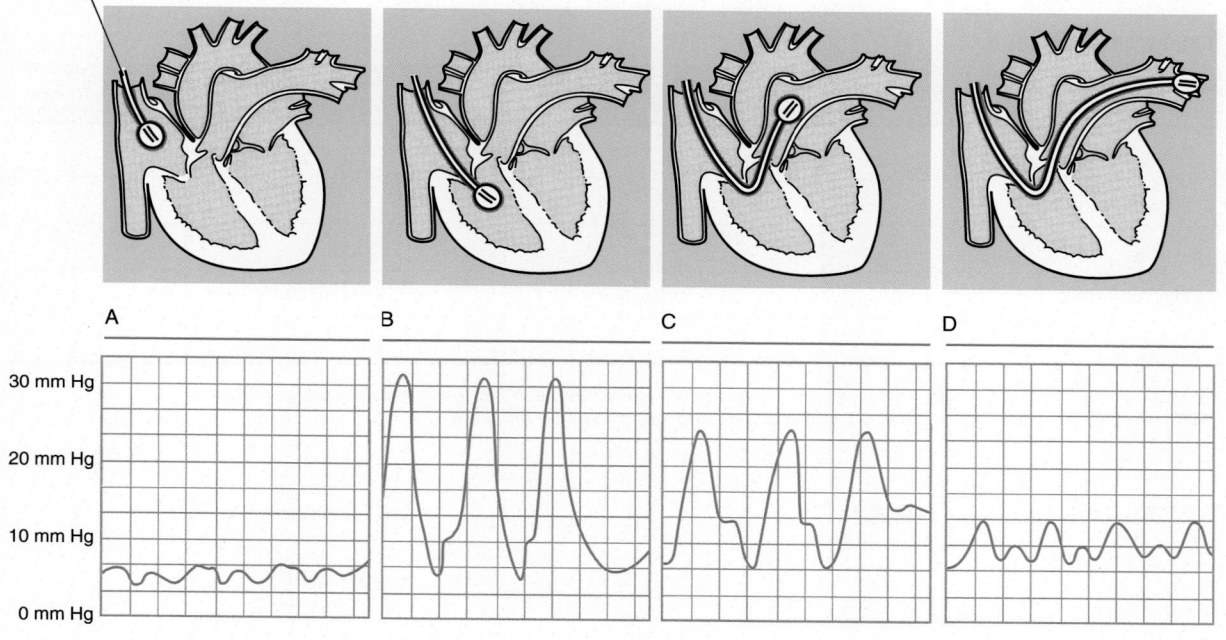

Flow-directed catheter

A   B   C   D

30 mm Hg

20 mm Hg

10 mm Hg

0 mm Hg

Exercise 2

Fill in the normal values for the following hemodynamic parameters.

Normal Values for the Hemodynamic Parameters

HEMODYNAMIC PARAMETER	NORMAL VALUE	INDICATES
HR		
CO		
RAP or CVP		
PAWP or PAOP		
PAP	Systolic:	
	Diastolic:	
SVR		
PVR		

HR, Heart rate; *CO,* cardiac output; *RAP,* right atrial pressure; *CVP,* central venous pressure; *PAWP,* pulmonary artery wedge pressure; *PAOP,* pulmonary artery occlusion pressure; *PAP,* pulmonary artery pressure; *SVR,* systemic vascular resistance; *PVR,* pulmonary vascular resistance.

Exercise 3

Insert an (↑) increase or decrease (↓) arrow in the following columns to indicate the hemodynamic value in each condition.

Hemodynamic Values

TYPES OF SHOCK	RAP	RVP	PAP	PAWP OR PAOP	CO	SVR
Anaphylactic						
Neurogenic						
Septic						
Hypovolemic						
Cardiogenic						

RAP, Right arterial pressure; *RVP,* right ventral pressure; *PAP,* pulmonary artery pressure; *PAWP,* pulmonary artery wedge pressure; *PAOP,* pulmonary artery occlusion pressure; *CO,* cardiac output; *SVR,* systemic vascular resistance.

1. What are the stages of shock?

   _____

   _____

   _____

2. Define the types of shock. (*If needed, include extra paper for longer definitions.*)

Anaphylactic _____

Neurogenic _____

Septic _____

Hypovolemic _____

Cardiogenic _____

Exercise 4

Insert an increase (↑) or decrease (↓) arrow in the following columns to indicate the major effect each drug or therapy has on the hemodynamic parameters listed. In the last column, list other benefits and potential side effects.

Effect Drugs and Therapy have on Hemodynamic Parameters

DRUG	HR	CO	SVR (AFTERLOAD)	PAWP/PAOP (PRELOAD)	BENEFITS AND POTENTIAL SIDE EFFECTS
Dobutamine					
Isoproterenol (Isuprel)					
Epinephrine					
Dopamine					
Sodium nitroprusside (Nipride)					
Nitroglycerin					
Norepinephrine (Levophed)					
Phenylephrine (Neo-Synephrine)					
Intraaortic balloon pump					
Morphine					
Lasix					
Phosphodiesterase inhibitors (Milrinone, Amrinone)					

HR, Heart rate; *RVP*, right ventral pressure; *CO*, cardiac output; *SVR*, systemic vascular resistance; *PAWP*, pulmonary artery wedge pressure; *PAOP*, pulmonary artery occlusion pressure.

Case Study 1

A 62-year-old man is admitted to the coronary care unit. On admission, he is complaining of chest pain and shortness of breath. Physical assessment reveals bibasilar crackles on auscultation, diaphoresis, poor capillary refill (greater than 3 seconds), and weak, thready pulses. His 12-lead electrocardiogram (ECG) shows that he has had an inferior wall myocardial infarction (MI) with significant Q waves in leads II, III, and aVF along with ST segment elevation. Chest radiograph shows bilateral infiltrates. Pulse oxime-try: Oxygen saturation is 85%, despite delivering 100% inspired oxygen (FIO_2). A pulmonary artery (PA) catheter is inserted.

Hemodynamic values are as follows:

- Heart rate (HR): 130 beats per minute (bpm)
- Respiratory rate: 32 breaths per minute
- Blood pressure (BP): 100/60 mm Hg
- CO: 2.8 L/min
- Cardiac index (CI): 1.2 L/min
- SVR: 1657 dynes/sec/cm^{-5}
- Right atrial pressure (RAP) or central venous pressure (CVP): 15 mm Hg
- Pulmonary artery wedge pressure (PAWP) or PAOP: 25 mm Hg

1. What is your interpretation of the hemodynamic values? (*If needed, include extra paper for a longer answer.*)

   _____

   _____

   _____

2. What would be the most probable diagnosis? (*Circle your answer.*)
   a. Left-sided heart failure
   b. Right-sided heart failure
   c. Adult respiratory distress syndrome
   d. Pneumonia with sepsis

3. Discuss the probable interventions. (*If needed, include extra paper for a longer answer.*)

   _____

   _____

   _____

   _____

   _____

Case Study 2

A 74-year-old man is admitted to the intensive care unit (ICU) with hypotension. He is not responsive but is breathing spontaneously. Urinary output is 50 ml in 6 hours. Breath sounds are clear and skin is cool. A PA catheter is inserted, and the following hemodynamic parameters have been obtained:

- BP: 88/50 mm Hg
- HR: 135 bpm
- Respiratory rate: 28/min
- Temperature: 37° C
- CVP: 2 mm Hg
- PAOP/PAWP: 4 mm Hg
- CO: 3 L/min
- PAP: 22/8 mm Hg
- Mixed venous oxygen saturation (SvO_2): 48%

1. How would you interpret these data?

_____

_____

_____

_____

_____

Case Study 3

Ms. JB was admitted to the ICU from a nursing home after having a large amount of coffee ground emesis. Her level of consciousness is decreased. A central line was placed. A Foley catheter was placed, and her urinary output for the first hour was 15 ml.

Her vital signs are as follows:

- BP: 86/44
- HR: 120 bpm
- Respiratory rate: 24/min
- Arterial oxygen saturation (SaO_2): 90% on room air
- CVP: 1 mm Hg

1. How would you interpret these data?

_____

_____

2. What would be an immediate consideration for Ms. JB?

_____

_____

_____

Case Study 4

A 56-year-old, 70-kg woman has been doing well 2 days after a colon resection. On the third day she feels more lethargic, and during the night she becomes confused and disoriented. Her vital signs show a temperature of 39° C, a pulse of 130/min, respirations of 28/min, and BP of 80/50 mm Hg. Her skin is flushed and her surgical wound site is reddened but has no drainage. Her lungs are clear. Pulse oximetry shows a saturation of 97%.

1. What therapeutic intervention should be performed first?

_____

_____

She receives a fluid bolus of 250 ml normal saline (NS) over 15 minutes. Her BP increases slightly to 82/52 mm Hg. A decision is made to transfer her to ICU and insert a PA catheter. Hemodynamic data obtained during PA catheter insertion include:

- CVP: 1 mm Hg
- PA: 25/10 mm Hg
- PAOP/PAWP: 8 mm Hg

2. Do these data determine the cause of her hypotension?

_____

_____

Next, the following values are obtained:
- CO: 12.5 L/min
- CI: 6.3 L/min
- SVR: 358 dynes/sec/cm^{-5}
- SvO$_2$: 85%

3. What do these data tell about the cause of her hypotension?

_____

_____

_____

_____

_____

_____

4. How should this condition be treated?

_____

_____

Case Study 5

A 56-year-old male comes into the emergency department with shortness of breath and extreme dyspnea on exertion. He has a history of a large anterior MI 6 months ago. His vital signs (VS) are an HR of 120/min, a respiration rate (RR) of 28/min, and BP of 180/110 mm Hg. A third heart sound is heard, and lung crackles are present bilaterally. He is placed on supplemental oxygen. He does not respond to a dose of 80-mg furosemide. He is admitted to the ICU with a diagnosis of heart failure.

A PA catheter is inserted, and the following data are obtained:
- CO: 3.3 L/min
- CI: 2.1 L/min
- SVR: 2690 dynes/sec/cm^{-5}

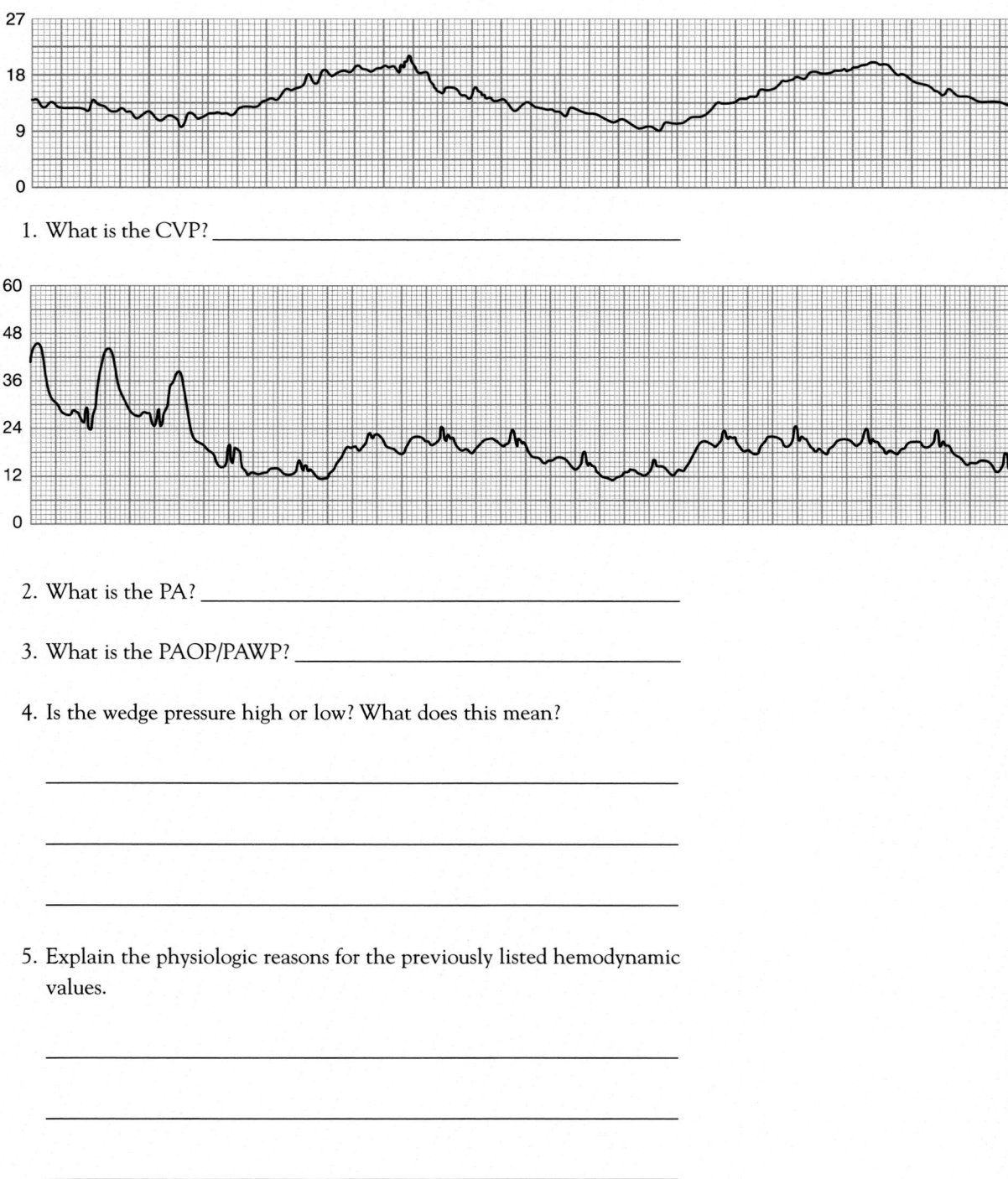

1. What is the CVP? _____

2. What is the PA? _____

3. What is the PAOP/PAWP? _____

4. Is the wedge pressure high or low? What does this mean?

   _____

   _____

   _____

5. Explain the physiologic reasons for the previously listed hemodynamic values.

   _____

   _____

   _____

6. What are the goals of treatment for this patient?

a. _____

b. _____

c. _____

A second dose of furosemide is given and a nesiritide (Natrecor) infusion begun. Urine output increases and respiratory distress improves. The following hemodynamic data are obtained:
- PAOP/PAWP: 12 mm Hg
- CO: 4.9 L/min
- CI: 3.5 L/min
- SVR: 1480 dynes/sec/cm^{-5}

7. Explain the differences in the hemodynamic values.

_____

_____

Case Study 6

A 38-year-old man is admitted to ICU after an episode of general fatigue, fever, and hypotension. He has been neutropenic secondary to chemotherapy. His HR is 140 bpm. His BP is 90/48 mm Hg. A PA catheter is inserted, and the following values obtained:
- PAOP/PAWP: 4 mm Hg
- CVP: 2 mm Hg
- CO: 12.5 L/min
- CI: 6.3 L/min
- SVR: 384 dynes/sec/cm^{-5}

1. Which of the following therapeutic interventions is most appropriate for this patient? (*Circle your answer.*)
   a. Fluid resuscitation, antibiotics, vasopressors
   b. Diuretics, positive inotropes
   c. Intraaortic balloon pump, sodium nitroprusside
   d. Beta blockers, calcium channel blockers

Case Study 7

An obese 45-year-old truck driver with a history of sleep apnea is admitted to ICU with symptoms of severe right-sided heart failure. A PA catheter is inserted and the following values obtained:

- Pulmonary artery pressures (PAS/PAD): 90/40 mm Hg
- PAOP/PAWP: 12 mm Hg
- CO: 6 L/min
- SVR: 880 dynes/sec/cm^{-5}
- Pulmonary vascular resistance (PVR): 400 dynes/sec/cm^{-5} (normal is less than 250 dynes/sec/cm^{-5})

1. These values suggest that the cause of his right-sided heart failure is what? *(Circle your answer.)*
   a. Left-sided heart failure
   b. Pulmonary hypertension
   c. Mitral regurgitation
   d. Sepsis

Solutions for Chapter 11: Clinical Application: Interventions, Exercises, & Case Studies

Exercise 1

A. Right atrial or CVP waveform
B. Right ventricular waveform
C. PA waveform
D. PA wedge waveform

Exercise 2

Normal Values for the Hemodynamic Parameters

HEMODYNAMIC PARAMETER	NORMAL VALUE	INDICATES
HR	60-100 beats/min	
CO	4-8 L/min	Amount of blood ejected by heart in 1 minute (SV × HR)
RAP or CVP	2-8 mm Hg	Right ventricular preload
PAWP or PAOP	6-12 mm Hg	Left ventricular preload
PAP	Systolic: 15-30 mm Hg	
	Diastolic: 6-12 mm Hg	
SVR	800-1200 dynes/sec/cm^{-5}	Left ventricular afterload
PVR	<250 dynes/sec/cm^{-5}	Right ventricular afterload

HR, Heart rate; *CO,* cardiac output; *RAP,* right atrial pressure; *CVP,* central venous pressure; *PAWP,* pulmonary artery wedge pressure; *PAOP,* pulmonary artery occlusion pressure; *PAP,* pulmonary artery pressure; *SVR,* systemic vascular resistance; *PVR,* pulmonary vascular resistance.

Exercise 3

Hemodynamic Values

TYPES OF SHOCK	RAP	RVP	PAP	PAWP OR PAOP	CO	SVR
Anaphylactic	↓	↓	↓	↓	↓	↓
Neurogenic	↓	↓	↓	↓	↓	↓
Septic	↓ ↑	↓	↓	↓	↑ ↓	↓ ↑
Hypovolemic	↓	↓	↓	↓	↓	↓
Cardiogenic	↑	↑	↑	↑	↓	↑

RAP, Right arterial pressure; *RVP,* right ventral pressure; *PAP,* pulmonary artery pressure; *PAWP,* pulmonary artery wedge pressure; *PAOP,* pulmonary artery occlusion pressure; *CO,* cardiac output; *SVR,* systemic vascular resistance.

1. Shock

- **Shock** is inadequate tissue perfusion, resulting in cellular hypoxia and dysfunction. The initial stage of shock is called the *compensatory stage*, during which vital organ perfusion is maintained through a complex series of neural, hormonal, and chemical responses. In the *progressive stage* of shock, impaired cellular function, altered systemic circulation, and altered capillary dynamics lead to multisystem organ failure. In the *refractory stage* of shock, heart failure, cerebral ischemia, acidosis, and coagulopathies result in death.

2. Types of Shock

- **Anaphylactic shock** is reduced tissue perfusion and hypotension, resulting from a specific antigen-antibody reaction. In this type of shock, histamine is released, which results in vasodilation, decreased SVR, and decreased BP. Serotonin is also released, which causes capillary leaks and fluid loss. These mediators cause decreased preload and decreased CO.
- **Neurogenic shock** results from loss of sympathetic tone, which causes bradycardia, vasodilation, and decreased BP, preload, and CO.
- **Septic shock** results from an overwhelming infection, which causes a systemic inflammatory response. The most common organisms are gram-negative bacteria, but viruses, fungi, or gram-positive organisms can also be causative factors.

Newer definitions for sepsis-related clinical conditions include:

Systemic inflammatory response syndrome (SIRS): Response to an insult or injury, independent of cause, with temperature elevations greater than 101.4° F, HR greater than 90 beats/minute. Tachypnea (respiratory rate greater than 20 breaths per minute or hyperventilation as indicated by a $PaCO_2$ less than 32 mm Hg, and a change in white blood cell count greater than 12,000 cells/mm³ or less than 4,000 cells/mm³).

Severe sepsis: Sepsis associated with hypotension, hypoperfusion, or signs of at least one acute organ dysfunction.

Shock: Sepsis-induced hypotension that persists despite adequate fluid resuscitation.

The cell wall of gram-negative organisms contain endotoxins that, when released, cause an inflammatory response, vasodilation, and increased capillary permeability. Fluid and protein leak from the intravascular compartment into the tissues results in decreased circulating volumes and decreased BP. In hyperdynamic septic shock the SVR is decreased and CO is increased. In hypodynamic septic shock, an increase in SVR and a decrease in CO both occur.

Anaphylactic, neurogenic, and septic shock are all forms of *distributive shock*. Fluid replacement is given for decreased preload. If afterload is decreased, then vasopressors are given. If afterload is increased, then vasodilators are given.

Hypovolemic shock occurs from massive intravascular volume loss, which results in decreased BP, preload, and CO. Interventions for hypovolemic shock include vasopressors and volume replacement.

Cardiogenic shock results from the inability of the heart to pump efficiently enough to maintain a normal CO, causing hypotension and impaired tissue perfusion. LV pump failure causes a decreased CO, decreased BP, increased pulmonary capillary wedge pressure, increased HR, and increased SVR. As cardiac work increases, CO continues to decrease, resulting in further decline of hemodynamics. Interventions for cardiogenic shock include improving cardiac contractility, reducing preload, afterload, and myocardial oxygen demands.

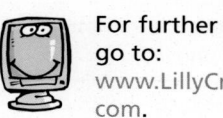

For further information go to:
www.LillyCriticalCare.com.

Exercise 4

Effect Drugs and Therapy have on Hemodynamic Parameters

DRUG	HR	CO	SVR (AFTERLOAD)	PAOP/PAWP (PRELOAD)	BENEFITS AND POTENTIAL SIDE EFFECTS
Dobutamine	↑	↑			Side effects: ↑ oxygen consumption potential for arrhythmias
Isoproterenol (Isuprel)	↑	↑			Side effects: ↑ oxygen consumption potential for arrhythmias
Epinephrine	↑	↑			Side effects: ↑ oxygen consumption potential for arrhythmias, peripheral ischemia
Dopamine		↑			Low dose is indicated for bradycardia or hypotensive patient Side effects: ↑ oxygen consumption potential for arrhythmias, peripheral ischemia
Sodium nitroprusside (Nipride)			↓	↓	Side effects: Cyanide toxicity hypotension
Nitroglycerin			↓	↓	Side effects: Headache, hypotension
Norepinephrine (Levophed)	↑		↑		Side effects: Peripheral ischemia
Phenylephrine (Neo-Synephrine)			↑		Side effects: Peripheral ischemia
Intraaortic balloon pump			↓		Improves coronary artery perfusion
Morphine			↓	↓	
Lasix				↓	
Phosphodiesterase inhibitors (Milrinone, Amrinone)					Increases contractility and promotes vasodilation; indicated for short-term treatment of heart failure patients who have not responded to vasodilators, diuretics, and digoxin

HR, Heart rate; *RVP,* right ventral pressure; *CO,* cardiac output; *SVR,* systemic vascular resistance; *PAWP,* pulmonary artery wedge pressure; *PAOP,* pulmonary artery occlusion pressure.

Case Study 1

1. The HR, respiratory rate, SVR, CVP, and PAWP are elevated.

2. A The clinical picture supports left-sided heart failure. The PAWP/PAOP (or left ventricular end–diastolic pressure) is elevated, reflecting the increased workload of the left ventricle secondary of fluid overload. The CVP is elevated directly as a result of increased volume. The CO is decreased because the heart cannot adequately pump this increased volume. The CVP is high to compensate for the decreased CO. This, in turn, decreased the CO even more because it creates more resistance to pumping.

   The clinical picture and hemodynamic values are not congruent with right-sided heart failure. Although the symptoms may be similar with severe refractory hypoxemia, acute respiratory distress syndrome is due to noncardiac pulmonary edema; therefore the PAWP/PAOP (left ventricular end–diastolic pressure) will not be elevated. The clinical picture does not match pneumonia. In addition, with sepsis, the CVP would be low and the BP would be low secondary to decreased volume.

3. Interventions would include diuretics and nitroglycerin (a venous dilator) for preload reduction and coronary artery perfusion, arteriolar dilators (e.g., nitroprusside to reduce SVR), and positive inotropic agents (e.g., dobutamine to increase contractility of the heart). In addition, oxygen saturation is maintained with supplemental oxygen via a delivery device that is effective.

Case Study 2

1. The CVP and CO are low, indicating low blood flow. The PAWP/PAOP is also low, which is consistent with hypovolemia. The low SvO_2 along with the decreased BP indicates a shock state as a result of decreased tissue oxygenation. The increased HR is a compensatory attempt to improve CO. Potential causes of the hypovolemia need to be considered, which would include gastrointestinal bleeding, dehydration, or other potential forms of blood loss.

Case Study 3

1. Ms. JB's CVP indicates hypovolemia. Her hypotension and tachycardia supports low volume status related to a probable gastrointestinal bleed.

2. A fluid bolus would be initially indicated for BP and volume improvement, which should reduce her HR. Ms. JB would need to be reassessed after the fluid bolus for any additional vasopressor drugs to improve BP. In addition, the source of the coffee ground emesis needs to be evaluated.

Case Study 4

1. Administer a fluid bolus. She is exhibiting signs of shock.
2. Not really. The CVP and PAWP/PAOP are low, suggesting that she is hypovolemic. However, the cause is unknown.
3. The CO and CI are very high. The SVR is low. Based on these data and her fever and recent surgery, systemic inflammatory response is leading to septic shock. The release of toxins in her bloodstream causes the blood vessel walls to dilate and seep fluid out, developing a "relative" hypovolemia. Her SVR reflects this massive vasodilation. Her CO is high because the heart is pumping hard to keep the blood vessels filled with blood to perfuse her vital organs. The increased metabolic needs of the body as a result of the febrile state also places demands on the heart to beat harder. Her SvO_2 is elevated because of the body's attempt to increase oxygen delivery, which is also due to the hyperdynamic state.
4. Treatment includes massive fluid resuscitation to "fill up the vascular space," as well as vasopressors such as dopamine or norepinephrine. Appropriate antibiotics should also be given.

Case Study 5

1. CVP: 20 mm Hg
2. PA: 40/24 mm Hg
3. PAWP/PAOP: 24 mm Hg
4. The PAWP/PAOP is elevated because he is in heart failure, which is leading to fluid backup in the lungs. The PAWP/PAOP is a reflection of the left atrial pressure and indirectly the left ventricular end–diastolic pressure. Elevation of the PAWP/PAOP is commonly observed in heart failure.
5. The CO and CI are low because the heart is failing. The SVR is high because the peripheral arterioles are vasoconstricting to keep the BP up as the heart fails.
6. The goals of treatment for this patient are to
   (a) Increase the contractility of the heart
   (b) Decrease the volume of blood returning to the heart (preload or PAWP/PAOP)
   (c) Decrease the peripheral resistance (afterload or SVR)
7. The nesiritide infusion has been successful in reducing preload; therefore the PAWP/PAOP has improved. The decrease in the SVR shows that less vasoconstriction now exists. Because the heart is not having to pump against so much resistance, the CO and CI have also increased.

Case Study 6

1. A This is the hemodynamic profile of sepsis. The SVR is decreased as a result of massive vasodilation from bacterial endotoxin. The CO is elevated because of a compensatory sympathetic response to attempt to fill up the large vascular space. The PAWP/PAOP is low because of a relative hypovolemia secondary to the vasodilation. Fluid is needed to fill up the vascular space; antibiotics are needed to fight the overwhelming infection; and vasopressors are given to "tighten up the space" to keep the blood pumping. Diuretics and positive inotropes would be contraindicated; they are more appropriate for heart failure. The intraaortic balloon pump and Nipride both decrease the SVR, which would be contraindicated in this case. Although beta-blockers and calcium channel-blockers decrease myocardial contractility and although this patient's contractility is high, this contractility is a necessary compensatory response and should not be suppressed.

Case Study 7

1. B The elevated pulmonary vascular resistance and PA pressures reflect massive pulmonary vasoconstriction and hypertension, probably a result of years of hypoxemia from sleep apnea. Although left-sided heart failure is the most common cause of right-sided failure, his PAWP/PAOP is normal, which suggests that his LV pressures are normal. Mitral regurgitation causes left-sided failure, not right. CO would be elevated, and SVR would be low in sepsis.

Appendix A

Esophageal Doppler Monitoring

Esophageal Doppler monitoring (EDM) works on the same Doppler principle that meteorologists use to warn of advancing severe weather or that traffic police use to stop speeding motorists. This principle states the following: the sound pitch of an object moving toward a receiver increases in frequency, whereas the sound pitch moving away from a receiver decreases in frequency. In the body, the Doppler principle is used to measure the velocity of red blood cells.

In EDM a pencil-thin ultrasound probe is lubricated, placed into the esophagus, and advanced to a location posterior to the heart at approximately the level of T5 to T6. The angled tip of the probe is oriented toward the descending aorta. The probe directs a beam of ultrasonic waves at the red blood cells and detects the speed of blood as it leaves the heart and travels through the descending aorta. The pulsatile blood flow produces a two-dimensional (velocity and time) physiologic waveform. Hemodynamic variables, such as cardiac output, preload, afterload, and contractility, are measured or derived from the EDM waveform.

When used in the surgical department, EDM can rapidly diagnose hemodynamic changes in patients with complex medical problems. It is especially useful in detecting significant blood loss or extensive fluid shifts. Because it is less invasive, has a low risk, and is as accurate as the pulmonary artery catheter, its use is expanding to critical care units and emergency departments.

EDM is contraindicated in patients with coarctation of the aorta, pathologic conditions of the esophagus, or intraaortic balloon pumps.

To learn more about the equipment needed for EDM, visit one of the following web sites:

 www.deltexmedical.com
www.hemosonic.com

Appendix B

Normal Hemodynamic Values

PARAMETERS MONITORED	HEMODYNAMIC FORMULAS	NORMAL VALUES
MAP	Systolic BP−diastolic BP ÷ 3 + diastolic BP	80-100 mm Hg Minimal acceptable MAP greater than or equal to 60 mm Hg
RAP/CVP RVP		0-8 mm Hg (Mean: 4 mm Hg) 15-30 mm Hg 0-8

Pulmonary artery pressures:
  PAS
  PAD
Pulmonary artery mean
PCWP/PAOP
		15-30 mm Hg
		6-12 mm Hg
		10-20 mm Hg
		4-12 mm Hg

CO	HR × SV	4-8 L/min
CI	CO ÷ BSA	2.5-4.0 L/min/m^2
SV	CO ÷ HR × 1000	60-130 ml/beat
SVI	CI × 1000 ÷ HR	333-347 ml/beat/m^2
LVSWI	(MAP−PCWP) × SVI × 0.0136	35-85 g/m^2/beat
RVSWI	(MPAP−RAP) × SVI × 0.0136	7-12 g/m^2/beat
SVR	(MAP−CVP) ÷ CO × 80	800-1400 dynes/sec/cm^5
SVRI	(MAP−CVP) ÷ CI × 80	1970-2390 dynes/sec/cm^5/m^2
PVR	(MPAP−PCWP) ÷ CO × 80	Less than 250 dynes/sec/cm^5
PVRI	(MPAP−PCWP) ÷ CI × 80	255-285 dynes/sec/cm^5/m^2
RVEF	RVSV ÷ RVEDV	40%-60%
LVEF	LVSV ÷ LVEDV	60%-70%

MAP, Mean arterial pressure; *BP,* blood pressure; *RAP,* right atrial pressure; *CVP,* central venous pressure; *RVP,* right ventricular pressure; *PAS,* pulmonary artery systolic; *PAD,* pulmonary artery diastolic; *PCWP,* pulmonary capillary wedge pressure; *PAOP,* pulmonary artery occlusion pressure; *CO,* cardiac output; *HR,* heart rate; *SV,* stroke volume; *CI,* cardiac index; *BSA,* body surface area; *SVI,* stroke volume index; *LVSWI,* left ventricular stroke work index; *RVSWI,* right ventricular stroke work index; *MPAP,* mean pulmonary arterial pressure; *SVR,* systemic vascular resistance; *SVRI,* systemic vascular resistance index; *PVR,* pulmonary vascular resistance; *PVRI,* pulmonary vascular resistance index; *RVEF,* right ventricular ejection fraction; *RVSV,* right ventricular stroke volume; *RVEDV,* right ventricular end–diastolic volume; *LVEF,* left ventricular ejection fraction; *LVSV,* left ventricular stroke volume; *LVEDV,* left ventricular end–diastolic volume.

Assessment of Oxygenation

PARAMETERS MONITORED	HEMODYNAMIC FORMULAS	NORMAL VALUES
CaO_2	Hgb × 1.34 × SaO_2	20 ml/dl
CvO_2	(Hgb × 1.34 × SvO_2) + (PvO_2 × 0.0031)	15 ml/dl
SaO_2		95%-100%
DO_2	CO × CaO_2 × 10 CO × (Hgb × 1.34 × SaO_2) × 10	1000ml/min Range: 640-1400 ml/min
VO_2	(CaO_2−CvO_2) × CO × 10	180-280 ml/min
SvO_2	Direct measurement	60%-80%

CaO_2, Arterial oxygen content; *Hgb,* hemoglobin; *CvO_2,* venous oxygen content; *SvO_2,* mixed venous oxygen saturation; *PvO_2,* mixed venous oxygen tension; *SaO_2,* arterial oxygen saturation; *DO_2,* oxygen delivery; *CO,* cardiac output; *VO_2,* oxygen consumption.

References

Chapter 1 Understanding the Heart & Lungs

Alspach JG et al: *AACN core curriculum for critical care nursing*, ed 5, Philadelphia, 1998, WB Saunders.

Darovic GO: *Hemodynamic monitoring: invasive and noninvasive clinical application*, ed 3, Philadelphia, 2002, WB Saunders.

Darovic GO, Franklin CM: *Handbook of hemodynamic monitoring*, Philadelphia, 1999, WB Saunders.

George-Gay B, Chernecky C: *Clinical medical-surgical nursing: a decision-making reference*, Philadelphia, 2002, WB Saunders.

Gutierrez KJ, Peterson PJ: *Real-world nursing survival guide: pathophysiology*, Philadelphia, 2002, WB Saunders.

Parsons PE, Wiener-Kronish JP: *Critical care secrets*, ed 2, Philadelphia, 2001, Hanley & Belfus.

Sole ML, Lamborn ML, Hartshorn JC: *Introduction to critical care nursing*, ed 3, Philadelphia, 2001, WB Saunders.

Chapter 2 Hemodynamic Theory

Alspach JG et al: *AACN core curriculum for critical care nursing*, ed 5, Philadelphia, 1998, WB Saunders.

Darovic GO: *Hemodynamic monitoring: invasive and noninvasive clinical application*, ed 3, Philadelphia, 2002, WB Saunders.

Darovic GO, Franklin CM: *Handbook of hemodynamic monitoring*, Philadelphia, 1999, WB Saunders.

George-Gay B, Chernecky C: *Clinical medical-surgical nursing: a decision-making reference*, Philadelphia, 2002, WB Saunders.

Gutierrez KJ, Peterson PJ: *Real-world nursing survival guide: pathophysiology*, Philadelphia, 2002, WB Saunders.

National Heart, Lung and Blood Institute, National Institute of Health: www.nhlbi.nih.gov/guidelines/hypertension. Reference card from the seventh report of the joint national committee on prevention, detection, evaluation and treatment of high blood pressure (JNC 7).

Parsons PE, Wiener-Kronish JP: *Critical care secrets*, 2nd ed, Philadelphia, 2001, Hanley & Belfus.

Sole ML, Lamborn ML, Hartshorn JC: *Introduction to critical care nursing*, ed 3, Philadelphia, 2001, WB Saunders.

Chapter 3 Hemodynamic Monitoring Equipment

Ahrens TS, Taylor L: *Hemodynamic waveform analysis*, Philadelphia, 1992, WB Saunders.

Alspach JG et al: *AACN core curriculum for critical care nursing*, ed 5, Philadelphia, 1998, WB Saunders.

Chernecky C, Berger B: *Laboratory tests and diagnostic procedures*, ed 2, Philadelphia, 1997, WB Saunders.

Chernecky C et al: *Real-world nursing survival guide: ECGs & the heart*, Philadelphia, 2002, WB Saunders.

Darovic GO: *Hemodynamic monitoring: invasive and noninvasive clinical application*, ed 3, Philadelphia, 2002, WB Saunders.

George-Gay B, Chernecky C: *Clinical medical-surgical nursing: a decision-making reference*, Philadelphia, 2002, WB Saunders.

Gutierrez KJ, Peterson PJ: *Real-world nursing survival guide: pathophysiology*, Philadelphia, 2002, WB Saunders.

Parsons PE, Wiener-Kronish JP: *Critical care secrets*, ed 2, Philadelphia, 2001, Hanley & Belfus.

Sole ML, Lamborn ML, Hartshorn JC: *Introduction to critical care nursing*, ed 3, Philadelphia, 2001, WB Saunders.

Chapter 4 Arterial Pressure Monitoring

American Association of Critical Care Nurses: www.critical-care-nurse.org/aacn/jrnlccn.nsf (articles).

Darovic GO: *Hemodynamic monitoring: invasive and noninvasive clinical application*, ed 3, Philadelphia, 2002, WB Saunders.

McGhee BH, Bridges MEJ: Monitoring arterial blood pressure: what you may not know, *Crit Care Nurs* 22(2):60, 2002.

McGhee BH, Woods SL: Critical care nurses' knowledge of arterial pressure monitoring, *Am J Crit Care* 10(1):43, 2001.

Sole ML, Lamborn ML, Hartshorn JC: *Introduction to critical care nursing*, ed 3, Philadelphia, 2001, WB Saunders.

Chapter 5 Right Atrial & Central Venous Pressure Monitoring

Ahrens TS, Taylor L: *Hemodynamic waveform analysis*, Philadelphia, 1992, WB Saunders.

Alspach JG et al: *AACN core curriculum for critical care nursing*, ed 5, Philadelphia, 1998, WB Saunders.

Darovic GO: *Hemodynamic monitoring: invasive and noninvasive clinical application*, ed 3, Philadelphia, 2002, WB Saunders.

Sole ML, Lamborn ML, Hartshorn JC: *Introduction to critical care nursing*, ed 3, Philadelphia, 2001, WB Saunders.

Chapter 6 Pulmonary Artery Pressure Monitoring

Ahrens TS, Taylor L: *Hemodynamic waveform analysis*, Philadelphia, 1992, WB Saunders.

Alspach JG: *AACN core review for critical care nursing*, ed 5, Philadelphia, 1998, WB Saunders.

Alspach JG et al: *AACN core curriculum for critical care nursing*, ed 5, Philadelphia, 1998, WB Saunders.

American Association of Critical Care Nurses: *Pulmonary artery catheter education project*, Aliso Viejo, Calif, 2001, www.PACEP.org.

Baxter Edwards (formerly American Edwards): *Hemodynamic training manual*, Irvine, Calif, 1979, Edwards Lifesciences LLC.

Edwards Life Science Healthcare Corporation—Critical Care Division: *Quick guide to cardiopulmonary care*, Irvine, Calif, 1998, Edwards Lifesciences LLC.

Chulay M, Guzzetta C, Dossey B: *AACN handbook of critical care nursing*, Stamford, Conn, 1997, Appleton & Lange.

Daily DK, Schroeder JS: Techniques in hemodynamic monitoring, ed 5, St Louis, 1994, Mosby.

Darovic GO: *Hemodynamic monitoring: invasive and noninvasive clinical application*, ed 3, Philadelphia, 2002, WB Saunders.

Darovic GO, Franklin CM: *Handbook of hemodynamic monitoring*, Philadelphia, 1999, WB Saunders.

Druding MC: Integrating hemodynamic monitoring and physical assessment, part II, *Nursing* 29(8):32, 1999.

Grap MJ, Pettrey L, Thornby D: Hemodynamic monitoring: a comparison of research and practice, *Am J Crit Care* 6(6):452, 1997.

Headley JM: Invasive hemodynamic monitoring: applying advanced technologies, *Crit Care Nurs Q* 21(3):73, 1998.

Kinney MR et al: *AACN clinical reference for critical care nursing*, ed 4, St Louis, 1998, Mosby.

Lynn-McHale DJ, Carlson KK: *AACN procedure manual for critical care*, ed 4, Philadelphia, 2001, WB Saunders.

Vitello-Cicciu JM, O-Sullivan CK: Hemodynamic monitoring. In Hartshorn JC, Sole ML, Lamborn ML: *Introduction to critical care nursing*, ed 3, Philadelphia, 2001, WB Saunders.

Chapter 7 Pulmonary Artery Pressures and Waveforms

Ahrens TS, Taylor L: *Hemodynamic waveform analysis*, Philadelphia, 1992, WB Saunders.

Alspach JG: *AACN core review for critical care nursing*, ed 5, Philadelphia, 1998, WB Saunders.

Alspach JG et al: *AACN core curriculum for critical care nursing*, ed 5, Philadelphia, 1998, WB Saunders.

American Association of Critical Care Nurses: *Pulmonary artery catheter education project*, 2001, www.PACEP.org.

Baxter Edwards (formerly American Edwards): *Hemodynamic training manual*, 1979, Edwards Lifesciences LLC.

Chulay M, Guzzetta C, Dossey B: *AACN handbook of critical care nursing*, Stamford, Conn, 1997, Appleton & Lange.

Daily DK, Schroeder JS: *Techniques in hemodynamic monitoring*, ed 5, St Louis, 1994, Mosby.

Darovic GO: *Hemodynamic monitoring: invasive and noninvasive clinical application*, ed 3, Philadelphia, 2002, WB Saunders.

Darovic GO, Franklin CM: *Handbook of hemodynamic monitoring*, Philadelphia, 1999, WB Saunders.

Druding MC: Integrating hemodynamic monitoring and physical assessment, part II, *Nursing* 29(8):32, 1999.

Edwards Life Science Healthcare Corporation—Critical Care Division: *Quick guide to cardiopulmonary care*, 1998, Irvine, Calif, Edwards Lifesciences LLC.

Grap MJ, Pettrey L, Thornby D: Hemodynamic monitoring: a comparison of research and practice, *Am J Crit Care* 6(6):452, 1997.

Headley JM: Invasive hemodynamic monitoring: applying advanced technologies, *Crit Care Nurs Q* 21(3):73, 1998.

Headley JM: Invasive hemodynamic monitoring: physiological principles and clinical applications, Irvine, Calif, 2002, Edwards Lifesciences LLC.

Kinney MR et al: *AACN clinical reference for critical care nursing*, ed 4, St Louis, 1998, Mosby.

Lynn-McHale DJ, Carlson KK: *AACN procedure manual for critical care*, ed 4, Philadelphia, 2001, WB Saunders.

Vitello-Cicciu JM, O-Sullivan CK: Hemodynamic monitoring. In Hartshorn JC, Sole ML, Lamborn ML: *Introduction to critical care nursing*, ed 3, Philadelphia, 2001, WB Saunders.

Chapter 8 Cardiac Output Measurements & Hemodynamic Calculations

Ahrens TS, Taylor L: *Hemodynamic waveform analysis*, Philadelphia, 1992, WB Saunders.

Alspach JG: *AACN core review for critical care nursing*, ed 5, Philadelphia, 1998, WB Saunders.

Alspach JG et al: *AACN core curriculum for critical care nursing*, ed 5, Philadelphia, 1998, WB Saunders.

American Association of Critical Care Nurses: *Pulmonary artery catheter education project*, 2001, www.PACEP.org.

Chulay M, Guzzetta C, Dossey B: *AACN handbook of critical care nursing*, Stamford, Conn, 1997, Appleton & Lange.

Daily DK, Schroeder JS: *Techniques in hemodynamic monitoring*, ed 5, St Louis, 1994, Mosby.

Darovic GO: *Hemodynamic monitoring: invasive and noninvasive clinical application*, ed 3, Philadelphia, 2002, WB Saunders.

Darovic GO, Franklin CM: *Handbook of hemodynamic monitoring*, Philadelphia, 1999, WB Saunders.

Druding MC: Integrating hemodynamic monitoring and physical assessment, part II, *Nursing* 29(8):32, 1999.

Edwards Life Science Healthcare Corporation—Critical Care Division: *Quick guide to cardiopulmonary care*, Irvine, Calif, 1998, Edwards Lifesciences LLC.

Grap MJ, Pettrey L, Thornby D: Hemodynamic monitoring: a comparison of research and practice, *Am J Crit Care* 6(6):452, 1997.

Headley JM: Invasive hemodynamic monitoring: applying advanced technologies, *Crit Care Nurs Q* 21(3):73, 1998.

Kinney MR et al: *AACN clinical reference for critical care nursing*, ed 4, St Louis, 1998, Mosby.

Lynn-McHale DJ, Carlson KK: *AACN procedure manual for critical care*, ed 4, Philadelphia, 2001, WB Saunders.

Vitello-Cicciu JM, O-Sullivan CK: Hemodynamic monitoring. In Hartshorn JC, Sole ML, Lamborn ML: *Introduction to critical care nursing*, ed 3, Philadelphia, 2001, WB Saunders.

Chapter 9 Mixed Venous Oxygen Monitoring

Barash P, Cullen B, Stoelting R, editors: *Clinical anesthesia*, ed 2, Philadelphia, 1992, Lippincott.

Chulay M, Guzzetta C, Dossey B: *AACN handbook of critical care nursing*, Stamford, Conn, 1997, Appleton & Lange.

Guyton AC, Hall JE: *Textbook of medical physiology*, ed 10, Philadelphia, 2002, WB Saunders.

Hudak CM, Gallo BM, Morton PG: *Critical care nursing: a holistic approach*, ed 7, Philadelphia, 1998, Lippincott.

Nagelhout J, Zaglaniczny K: *Nurse anesthesia*, ed 2, Philadelphia, 2001, WB Saunders.

Skeehan TM, Thys DM: Monitoring the cardiac surgical patient. In Hensley F, Martin D, editor: *A practical approach to cardiac anesthesia*, ed 2, Boston, 1995, Little, Brown & Company.

Stoelting RK, Miller RD: *Basics of anesthesia*, ed 4, New York, 2000, Churchill Livingstone.

Chapter 10 Noninvasive Hemodynamic Monitoring

Arrow International: Reading, Penn, 2003, Hemosonic device, www.hemosonic.com.

Cardiodynamics International: San Diego, 2003, BioZ ICG device, www.cardiodynamics.com and www.impedancecardiography.com.

Deltex Medical, Chichester, UK, 2003 CardioQ hemodynamic monitoring system, www.deltexmedical.com.

Lasater M: *Impedance cardiography: a method of noninvasive cardiac output monitoring*, 2003, AACN's Continuing Education Website, www.aacn.org.

Turner MA: Doppler-based hemodynamic monitoring: a minimally invasive alternative, *AACN Clin Issues* 14(2):220, 2003.

Von Rueden KT, Turner MA, Lynn CA: A new approach to hemodynamic monitoring, *RN* 62(8):52, 1999.

Chapter 11 Clinical Applications

Ahrens TS, Taylor L: *Hemodynamic waveform analysis*, Philadelphia, 1992, WB Saunders.

Alspach JG: *AACN core review for critical care nursing*, ed 5, Philadelphia, 1998, WB Saunders.

Alspach JG et al: *AACN core curriculum for critical care nursing*, ed 5, Philadelphia, 1998, WB Saunders.

American Association of Critical Care Nurses: *Pulmonary artery catheter education project*, 2001, www.PACEP.org.

Chernecky C, Berger B: *Laboratory tests and diagnostic procedures*, ed 2, Philadelphia, 1997, WB Saunders.

Chernecky C et al: *Real-world nursing survival guide: ECGs & the heart*, Philadelphia, 2002, WB Saunders.

Chulay M, Guzzetta C, Dossey B: *AACN handbook of critical care nursing*, Stamford, Conn, 1997, Appleton & Lange.

Daily DK, Schroeder JS: *Techniques in hemodynamic monitoring*, ed 5, St Louis, 1994, Mosby.

Darovic GO: *Hemodynamic monitoring: invasive and noninvasive clinical application*, ed 3, Philadelphia, 2002, WB Saunders.

Darovic GO, Franklin CM: *Handbook of hemodynamic monitoring*, Philadelphia, 1999, WB Saunders.

Druding MC: Integrating hemodynamic monitoring and physical assessment, part II, *Nursing* 29(8):32, 1999.

Edwards Life Science Healthcare Corporation—Critical Care Division: *Quick guide to cardiopulmonary care*, Irvine, Calif, 1998, Edwards Lifesciences LLC.

George-Gay B, Chernecky C: *Clinical medical-surgical nursing: a decision making reference*, Philadelphia, 2002, WB Saunders.

Gutierrez KJ, Peterson PJ: *Real-world nursing survival guide: pathophysiology*, Philadelphia, 2002, WB Saunders.

Headley JM: Invasive hemodynamic monitoring: applying advanced technologies, *Crit Care Nurs Q* 21(3):73, 1998.

Kinney MR et al: *AACN clinical reference for critical care nursing*, ed 4, St Louis, 1998, Mosby.

Lewis SM, Heitkemper MM, Dirksen SR: *Medical-surgical nursing: assessment and management of clinical problems*, St Louis, 2000, Mosby.

Lynn-McHale DJ, Carlson KK: *AACN procedure manual for critical care*, ed 4, Philadelphia, 2001, WB Saunders.

Sole ML, Lamborn ML, Hartshorn JC: *Introduction to critical care nursing*, ed 3, Philadelphia, 2001, WB Saunders.

Vitello-Cicciu JM, O-Sullivan CK: Hemodynamic monitoring. In Hartshorn JC, Sole ML, Lamborn ML: *Introduction to critical care nursing*, ed 3, Philadelphia, 2001, WB Saunders.

Illustration Credits

Chapter 1 Understanding the Heart & Lungs

Page 4 Redrawn from Alspach J et al: *AACN core curriculum for critical care nursing*, ed 5, pg 147, Philadelphia, 1998, WB Saunders.

Page 7 Redrawn from Alspach J et al: *AACN core curriculum for critical care nursing*, ed 5, pg 143, Philadelphia, 1998, WB Saunders.

Page 8 Redrawn from Jarvis C: *Physical examination and health assessment*, ed 4, pg 488, Philadelphia, 2004, WB Saunders.

Page 12 Redrawn from Sole ML et al: *Introduction to critical care nursing*, ed 3, pg 118, Philadelphia, 2001, WB Saunders.

Page 13 Redrawn from Eubanks D, Bone RC: *Comprehensive respiratory care: a learning system*, ed 2, pg 168, St Louis, 1990, Mosby.

Page 14 Redrawn from Rushmer RF: *Organ physiology: structure and function of the cardiovascular system*, ed 2, Philadelphia, 1976, WB Saunders.

Chapter 2 Hemodynamic Theory

Page 19 Redrawn from Sole ML et al: *Introduction to critical care nursing*, ed 3, pg 102, Philadelphia, 2001, WB Saunders.

Page 22 Redrawn from Sole ML et al: *Introduction to critical care nursing*, ed 3, pg 89, Philadelphia, 2001, WB Saunders.

Page 30 Redrawn from Alspach J et al: *AACN core curriculum for critical care nursing*, ed 5, pg 193, Philadelphia, 1998, WB Saunders.

Page 31 Redrawn from Alspach J et al: *AACN core curriculum for critical care nursing*, ed 5, pg 194, Philadelphia, 1998, WB Saunders.

Page 33 Redrawn from Sole ML et al: *Introduction to critical care nursing*, ed 3, pg 90, Philadelphia, 2001, WB Saunders. From Jackie M, Halligan M: *Cardiovascular problems: a critical care nursing focus*, Bowie MD, Brady RJ.

Page 36 Redrawn from Sole ML et al: *Introduction to critical care nursing*, ed 3, pg 121, Philadelphia, 2001, WB Saunders. Modified from Alspach J: *AACN instructor's resource manual for the AACN core curriculum for critical care nursing (transparency 29)*, Philadelphia, 1992, WB Saunders.

Chapter 3 Hemodynamic Monitoring Equipment

Page 39 Redrawn from Darovic GO: *Hemodynamic monitoring, invasive and noninvasive clinical application*, ed 3, pg 196, Philadelphia, 2002, WB Saunders.

Page 41 Redrawn from Sole ML et al: *Introduction to critical care nursing*, ed 3, pg 101, Philadelphia, 2001, WB Saunders.

Page 42 Redrawn from Darovic GO: *Hemodynamic monitoring, invasive and noninvasive clinical application*, ed 3, pg 164. Philadelphia, 2002, WB Saunders.

Page 47 Redrawn from Sole ML et al: *Introduction to critical care nursing*, ed 3, pg 90, Philadelphia, 2001, WB Saunders.

Page 48 Redrawn from Darovic GO: *Hemodynamic monitoring, invasive and noninvasive clinical application*, ed 3, pg 128, Philadelphia, 2002, WB Saunders. From Gardner RM, Hollingsworth, KW: Optimizing the electrocardiogram and pressure monitoring, *Crit Care Med* 14: 651, 1986.

Page 52 (top) Redrawn from Darovic GO: *Hemodynamic monitoring, invasive and noninvasive clinical application*, ed 3, pg 122, Philadelphia, 2002, WB Saunders.

Page 52 (bottom) Redrawn from Darovic GO: *Hemodynamic monitoring, invasive and noninvasive clinical application*, ed 3, pg 122, Philadelphia, 2002, WB Saunders.

Page 54 Redrawn from Darovic GO: *Hemodynamic monitoring, invasive and noninvasive clinical application*, ed 3, pg 224, Philadelphia, 2002, WB Saunders.

Chapter 4 Arterial Pressure Monitoring

Pages 62-63 (Table) Modified from Darovic GO: *Hemodynamic monitoring, invasive and noninvasive clinical application*, ed 3, pgs 151-152, Philadelphia, 2002, WB Saunders.

Page 60 Redrawn from Sole ML et al: *Introduction to critical care nursing*, ed 3, pg 90, Philadelphia, 2001, WB Saunders.

Page 61 Redrawn from Bucher L, Melander SD: *Critical care nursing*, pg 120, Philadelphia, 1999, WB Saunders.

Page 65 Redrawn from Sole ML et al: *Introduction to critical care nursing*, ed 3, pg 93, Philadelphia, 2001, WB Saunders.

Page 66 Redrawn from Bucher L, Melander SD: *Critical care nursing*, pg 121, Philadelphia, 1999, WB Saunders.

Page 67 (top) Redrawn from Urden LD, Stacy KM, Lough ME: *Thelan's critical care nursing: diagnosis and management*, ed 4, pg 366, St Louis, 2002, Mosby.

Page 67 (bottom) Redrawn from Urden LD, Stacy KM, Lough ME: *Thelan's critical care nursing: diagnosis and management*, ed 4, pg 366, St Louis, 2002, Mosby.

Chapter 5 Right Atrial & Central Venous Pressure Monitoring

Page 75 Redrawn from Lewis SM et al: *Medical-surgical nursing: assessment and management of clinical problems*, ed 6, pg 1765, St Louis, 2003, Mosby. Redrawn from Flynn JBM, Bruce NP: *Introduction to critical care skills*, St Louis, 1993, Mosby.

Page 78 Redrawn from Boggs RL, Wooldridge-King M: *AACN procedure manual for critical care*, ed 3, pg 308, Philadelphia, 1993, WB Saunders.

Page 80 Redrawn from Alspach J et al: *AACN core curriculum for critical care nursing*, ed 5, pg 306, Philadelphia, 1998, WB Saunders. From Hudak: *Critical care nursing: a holistic approach*, pg 123, Philadelphia, 1989, Lippincott.

Chapter 6 Pulmonary Artery Pressure Monitoring

Page 91 Visalli F, Evans P: *Hemodynamic training manual: the Swan-Ganz catheter: a program for teaching safe, effective use*, Baxter Edwards Life Sciences, 1979.

Page 94 *Quick guide to pulmonary care*, 1998, Irvine, Calif, Edwards Lifesciences Co, 1998.

Page 97 Redrawn from Alspach J et al: *AACN core curriculum for critical care nursing*, ed 5, pg 194, Philadelphia, 1998, WB Saunders.

Page 98 Visalli F, Evans P: *Hemodynamic training manual: the Swan-Ganz catheter: a program for teaching safe, effective use*, Baxter Edwards Life Sciences, 1979.

Page 100 *Quick guide to pulmonary care*, 1998, Irvine, Calif, Edwards Lifesciences Co, 1998.

Chapter 7 Pulmonary Artery Pressures and Waveforms

Page 105 *(top)* Courtesy of Maureen Harvey, CCRN review course, 1982, Memphis, Tenn.

Page 105 *(bottom)* Redrawn from Daily EK: *Techniques in hemodynamics: monitoring waveforms*, St Louis, 1994, Mosby.

Page 107 Redrawn from Edwards Life Science Healthcare Corporation—Critical Care Division: *Quick guide to cardiopulmonary care*, 1998, Irvine, Calif, Edwards Lifesciences LLC.

Page 108 Redrawn from Alspach J et al: *AACN core curriculum for critical care nursing*, ed 5, pg 194, Philadelphia, 1998, WB Saunders.

Page 113 Redrawn from Daily EK: *Techniques in hemodynamics: monitoring waveforms*, St Louis, 1994, Mosby.

Page 115 Redrawn from Edwards Life Science Healthcare Corporation—Critical Care Division: *Quick guide to cardiopulmonary care*, 1998, Irvine, Calif, Edwards Lifesciences LLC.

Page 117 Baxter Edwards (formerly American Edwards): *Hemodynamic training manual*, 1979, Edwards Lifesciences LLC.

Page 120 Redrawn from Ahrens T, Taylor L: *Hemodynamic waveform analysis*, pg 170, Philadelphia, 1992, WB Saunders.

Page 121 Redrawn from Darovic GO: *Hemodynamic monitoring, invasive and noninvasive clinical application*, ed 3, pg 209, Philadelphia, 2002, WB Saunders.

Chapter 8 Cardiac Output Measurements & Hemodynamic Calculations

Page 122 Redrawn from Sole ML et al: *Introduction to critical care nursing*, ed 3, pg 89, Philadelphia, 2001, WB Saunders.

Page 123 Redrawn from Meschan I, Ott DJ: *Introduction to diagnostic imaging*, Philadelphia, 1984, WB Saunders.

Page 126 Redrawn from Darovic GO: *Hemodynamic monitoring, invasive and noninvasive clinical application*, ed 3, pg 252, Philadelphia, 2002, WB Saunders. Adapted from Marino PL: Thermodilution cardiac output. In Marino PL: *The ICU book*, Philadelphia, 1991, Lea & Febiger.

Page 127 Redrawn from Spacelabs Medical (operations manual), 1995.

Page 128 Redrawn from Spacelabs Medical, (operations manual), 1995.

Page 129 Redrawn from Darovic GO: *Hemodynamic monitoring, invasive and noninvasive clinical application*, ed 3, pg 252, Philadelphia, 2002, WB Saunders. Copyright © Hewlett-Packard Company. Reproduced with permission.

Chapter 9 Mixed Venous Oxygen Monitoring

Page 139 Redrawn from Alspach J et al: *AACN core curriculum for critical care nursing*, ed 5, pg 194, Philadelphia, 1998, WB Saunders.

Chapter 10 Noninvasive Hemodynamic Monitoring

Page 145 Redrawn from Darovic GO: *Hemodynamic monitoring, invasive and noninvasive clinical application*, ed 3, pg 252, Philadelphia, 2002, WB Saunders. Cardiodynamics International Corp, San Diego, Calif. Reprinted with permission.

Page 146 *(top)* Redrawn from Darovic GO: *Hemodynamic monitoring, invasive and noninvasive clinical application*, ed 3, pg 260, Philadelphia, 2002, WB Saunders. Cardiodynamics International Corp, San Diego, Calif. Reprinted with permission.

Page 146 *(bottom)* Redrawn from von Rueden KT: Noninvasive hemodynamic monitoring: impedance cardiography. In Lynn-McHale D, Carlson D: *AACN procedure manual for critical care*, ed 4, pg 421, Philadelphia, 2001, WB Saunders.

Chapter 11 Clinical Applications

Page 152 Redrawn from Lewis SM, Heitkemper MM, DirksenSR: *Medical-surgical nursing: assessment and management of clinical problems*, ed 5, pg 1923, St Louis, 2000, Mosby.

NCLEX® Examination Review Questions

Understanding the Heart and Lungs

1. If you were to trace a drop of blood from the venous system through the heart to the systemic circulation, blood would flow from
   1 the left ventricle and then to the pulmonary veins, lungs, and systemic circulation.
   2 the superior or inferior vena cava and then to the right atrium, right ventricle, pulmonary artery, lungs (pulmonary capillary bed), pulmonary veins, left atrium, left ventricle, aorta, and systemic circulation.
   3 the right atrium and then to the right ventricle, pulmonary veins, lungs, pulmonary artery, left atrium, left ventricle, aorta, and systemic circulation.
   4 the left atrium and then to the right ventricle, lungs, right atrium, left ventricle, aorta, and systemic circulation.

2. The term used when the ventricles are contracting is
   1 systole.
   2 diastole.
   3 filling.
   4 resting.

3. Another name for filling of the ventricles is
   1 systole.
   2 diastole.
   3 contraction.
   4 ejection.

4. What chamber of the heart pumps blood into the pulmonary artery?
   1 Right atrium
   2 Right ventricle
   3 Left atrium
   4 Left ventricle

5. During diastole, which valves in the heart are open?
   1 Pulmonic and aortic
   2 Mitral and tricuspid
   3 Aortic and tricuspid
   4 Mitral and pulmonic

6. The electrical conduction system is the stimulus for ventricular
   1 filling.
   2 relaxation.
   3 contraction.
   4 diastole.

7. During diastole, a continuous open circuit in the heart exists from the
   1 tricuspid valve to the mitral valve.
   2 pulmonic valve to the aortic valve.
   3 aortic valve to the tricuspid valve.
   4 pulmonic valve to the mitral valve.

8. The amount of blood in the left ventricle before ejection is called
   1 left ventricular–end systolic volume.
   2 left ventricular–end diastolic volume.
   3 ejection fraction.
   4 stroke volume.

9. The movement of respiratory gas molecules across cell membranes is called
   1 ventilation.
   2 respiration.
   3 distribution.
   4 inhalation.

CHAPTER *1*—cont'd

10. The pressure that the right ventricle must overcome to promote forward flow of blood through the pulmonary circulation is called
    1 systemic vascular resistance.
    2 distribution.
    3 pulmonary vascular resistance.
    4 coronary artery circulation.

CHAPTER *2*

Hemodynamic Theory

1. At the end of diastole, the degree of ventricular stretch is referred to as
    1 preload.
    2 afterload.
    3 contractility.
    4 cardiac output.

2. The cardiac conduction system is the stimulus for
    1 atrial filling.
    2 ventricular contraction.
    3 systemic vascular resistance.
    4 afterload.

3. The formula for cardiac output states that cardiac output equals
    1 stroke volume multiplied by heart rate.
    2 patient weight multiplied by heart rate.
    3 contractility multiplied by heart rate.
    4 stroke volume multiplied by contractility.

4. Which of the following is **not** a determinant of stroke volume?
    1 Contractility
    2 Preload
    3 Heart rate
    4 Afterload

5. Preload is
    1 a measurement of systemic vascular resistance.
    2 a measurement reflecting contractility.
    3 reflective of left ventricular-end diastolic volume.
    4 reflective of cardiac output.

6. Afterload is reflective of
    1 pulmonary capillary wedge pressure or PAOP.
    2 cardiac output.
    3 contractility.
    4 systemic vascular resistance.

CHAPTER 2—cont'd

7. A substance that affects contractility is referred to as
   1 chronotropic.
   2 inotropic.
   3 vasoactive.
   4 vasodilatory.

8. Preload can be measured with a pulmonary artery catheter by obtaining
   1 systemic vascular resistance.
   2 pulmonary capillary wedge pressure or PAOP.
   3 left ventricular stroke work index.
   4 pulmonary artery systolic pressure.

9. The sum of resistance in peripheral arterioles reflected in mean aortic pressure is
   1 pulmonary vascular resistance.
   2 systemic vascular resistance.
   3 mean arterial pressure.
   4 pulmonary capillary wedge pressure.

10. Miscellaneous influences that **decrease** contractility include
   1 hypoxia, hyperkalemia, and sympathetic stimulation.
   2 hypercarbia, hyponatremia, and sympathetic stimulation.
   3 hypoxia, myocardial scar tissue, and parasympathetic stimulation.
   4 hypokalemia, hypernatremia, and parasympathetic stimulation.

CHAPTER 3

Hemodynamic Monitoring Equipment

1. A pulmonary artery catheter can be used to monitor
   1 pulmonary artery systolic pressure only.
   2 arterial pressure, pulmonary artery systolic pressure, pulmonary artery diastolic pressure, and central venous pressure.
   3 pulmonary artery systolic pressure, pulmonary artery diastolic pressure, central venous pressure.
   4 arterial pressure and pulmonary artery diastolic pressure.

2. Potential complications of a pulmonary artery catheter include
   1 ventricular ectopy and pulmonary artery rupture.
   2 ventricular ectopy, pulmonary artery rupture, and emboli.
   3 heart blocks, pulmonary artery rupture, and emboli.
   4 ventricular ectopy, heart blocks, pulmonary artery rupture, and emboli.

3. The Allen's test is used to
   1 detect ischemia in the heart.
   2 determine hematocrit.
   3 determine oxygen consumption.
   4 detect appropriate collateral circulation in the ulnar artery.

4. Transducers used in hemodynamic monitoring should be leveled at the
   1 phlebostatic axis.
   2 left lower lung.
   3 right hand.
   4 right internal jugular vein.

5. To zero a transducer, the stopcock is
   1 closed to the air and opened to the patient.
   2 opened to the air and opened to the patient.
   3 opened to the air and closed to the patient.
   4 closed to the air and closed to the patient.

6. The test used to check the ability of the fluid-filled monitoring system to reproduce the patient's pressure accurately on the monitor is called
   1 Allen's.
   2 Schilling.
   3 ice water caloric.
   4 square wave.

7. The phlebostatic axis is located at the
   1 second intercostal space and midclavicular position.
   2 fourth intercostal space and midaxillary position.
   3 fifth intercostal space and anterior axillary position.
   4 fifth intercostal space and lower left sternal border.

CHAPTER *3*—cont'd

8. To obtain reliable hemodynamic measurements, you should
   1 ensure proper patient positioning, that the system is fluid filled and air-bubble free, and that all connections are tightened.
   2 level and zero the transducer, ensure proper patient positioning, that the system is fluid filled and air-bubble free, and that all connections are tightened.
   3 level and zero the transducer and ensure proper patient positioning.
   4 level and zero the transducer, ensure proper patient positioning, and ensure that the system is fluid filled and air-bubble free and that all connections are tightened.

9. The pressure bag on the flush solution should be inflated to
   1 300 mm Hg.
   2 250 mm Hg.
   3 200 mm Hg.
   4 350 mm Hg.

10. Patient preparation for hemodynamic monitoring includes
    1 washing hands only.
    2 washing hands, having emergency equipment available, explaining the procedure to the patient, and ensuring all consent forms are signed.
    3 having emergency equipment available and ensuring all consent forms are signed.
    4 washing hands, having emergency equipment available, and ensuring all consent forms are signed.

CHAPTER *4*

Arterial Pressure Monitoring

1. The use of an arterial pressure monitoring would be indicated for all of the following conditions *except*
   1 for the patient who is receiving sodium nitroprusside (Nipride) infusion.
   2 for the patient in hypovolemic shock who has a systolic blood pressure less than 85 mm Hg.
   3 to administer intravenous medications during an emergency.
   4 to draw frequent arterial blood gases and laboratory studies.

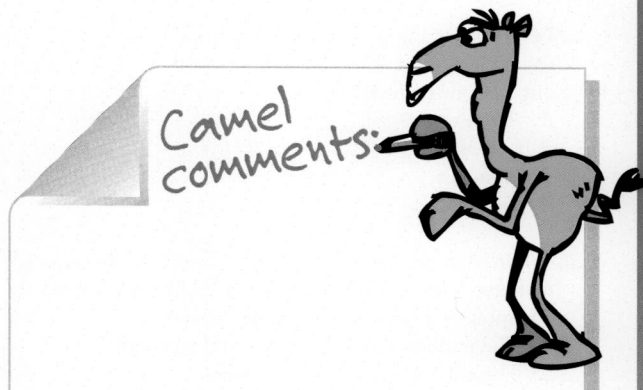

Camel comments:

CHAPTER *4*—cont'd

2. Before inserting a radial arterial line, a(n) _____ test should be performed to assess whether the collateral circulation is effective.
   1 Allen's
   2 Chvostek's
   3 Homan's
   4 Trousseau's

3. When determining the site for inserting an arterial catheter, which of the following would be considered an advantage for selecting the pedal artery?
   1 The patient will be able to stand and walk.
   2 Thrombotic occlusion is minimal.
   3 The patient has had numerous arterial lines in other sites.
   4 A less chance exists for monitor artifacts, and readings are very accurate.

4. Which of the following may overdamp the arterial pressure waveform of a radial catheter?
   1 Air bubbles
   2 Full flush bag
   3 Immobilization of the wrist
   4 Febrile state of patient

5. After inserting a right femoral arterial line, it is important to assess which of the following?
   1 Presence of abnormal heart sounds
   2 Ability of patient to feel and move the left foot
   3 Level of consciousness and bilateral pupil response
   4 Right foot color, temperature, and pedal pulse

6. The dicrotic notch on an arterial waveform tracing represents the closure of which of the following heart valves?
   1 Tricuspid
   2 Aortic
   3 Pulmonic
   4 Mitral

7. All of the following are possible complications that can occur from an arterial line *except*
   1 infection.
   2 air embolism.
   3 increased extremity blood flow.
   4 exsanguination.

8. How long is it necessary to apply pressure on the arterial puncture site when the catheter is discontinued?
   1 1 minute
   2 2 to 3 minutes
   3 4 minutes
   4 5 to 10 minutes

9. Which of the following may underdamp the arterial pressure waveform?
   1 Six-foot tubing
   2 Numerous stopcocks
   3 Bent tubing
   4 Empty flush bag

10. Which of the following arterial sites is the site where pressure is released to determine the results of the Allen's test?
    1 Axillary
    2 Brachial
    3 Radial
    4 Ulnar

CHAPTER *5*

Right Atrial and Central Venous Pressure Monitoring

1. Central venous pressure correlates most directly with
   1 left ventricular pressure.
   2 right atrial pressure.
   3 right ventricular pressure.
   4 left atrial pressure.

2. Normal central venous pressure is from
   1 8 to 10 mm Hg.
   2 6 to 12 mm Hg.
   3 0 to 8 mm Hg.
   4 0 to 4 mm Hg.

3. During central venous pressure insertion, the role of the circulating nurse is to
   1 monitor and comfort the patient.
   2 assist the operating physician.
   3 gather supplies.
   4 watch the monitor.

CHAPTER *5*—cont'd

4. Ideally, central venous pressure should be measured with the patient
   1 at 45 degrees.
   2 on his or her left side.
   3 in a supine position of 30 degrees or less.
   4 in the Trendelenburg position.

5. With water manometer or transducer, the central venous pressure should be measured at the
   1 midaxillary line.
   2 intramammary line.
   3 level of the left ventricle.
   4 phlebostatic axis.

6. When measuring central venous pressure with a pressure transducer, the right atrial pressure is measured
   1 at the end of expiration.
   2 at the end of inspiration.
   3 at the beginning of inspiration.
   4 any time during the respiratory cycle.

7. A low central venous pressure may indicate
   1 fluid overload.
   2 hypovolemia.
   3 left heart failure.
   4 cardiac tamponade.

8. If the patient's central venous pressure reading is low, which of the following interventions may help determine whether the patient is hypovolemic?
   1 Providing continuous readings
   2 Measuring the central venous pressure with the patient on a ventilator
   3 Reading the central venous pressure with the patient in different positions
   4 Providing a fluid challenge

9. One of the most immediate life-threatening complications related to central venous catheters is
   1 infection.
   2 air embolus.
   3 hemorrhage.
   4 pneumothorax.

Camel comments:

CHAPTER *5*—cont'd

10. When removing a central venous catheter,
    1 minimal resistance should occur.
    2 some resistance is to be expected, especially if the catheter has been in for a prolonged time.
    3 apply steady pressure to remove the catheter if resistance is felt.
    4 apply stop and advance the catheter slightly if resistance is felt.

CHAPTER *6*

Pulmonary Artery Pressure Monitoring

1. Which of the following statements is **true** regarding the distal port of the pulmonary artery catheter?
    1 It is connected to a pressure transducer and a flush device.
    2 It is the port used for cardiac output injectate.
    3 It allows continuous measurement of pulmonary artery occlusive pressure.
    4 It serves as an infusion port for vasoactive medications.

2. The purpose of the venous infusion port on the Swan-Ganz catheter is to
    1 measure systemic vascular resistance.
    2 measure cardiac output.
    3 draw mixed venous gases.
    4 have an extra site for intravenous medication infusion.

3. During the insertion of a pulmonary artery catheter, when the tip is in the right atrium, how much air should be used to inflate the balloon?
    1 $^1/_2$ ml
    2 1 ml
    3 $1^1/_2$ ml
    4 2 ml

4. A pulmonary artery catheter is necessary to measure the three determinants of stroke volume. These are
    1 excitability, conductivity, and automaticity.
    2 preload, afterload, and contractility.
    3 heart rate, preload, and afterload.
    4 cardiac output, heart rate, and blood pressure.

5. The physiologic event that causes the appearance of the dicrotic notch on the pulmonary artery waveform is the
    1 opening of the aortic valve.
    2 closing of the aortic valve.
    3 opening of the pulmonic valve.
    4 closing of the pulmonic valve.

6. Which of the following statements about the technical aspects of pulmonary artery catheter insertion is **true?**
    1 The pressure cuff on the solution bag should be maintained at 200 mm Hg.
    2 The side port of the transducer should be leveled at the patient's right atrial level.
    3 The monitor should be set on a scale of 0 to 300 mm Hg.
    4 Vented caps should be placed on all stopcock ports.

7. The pulmonary artery systolic pressure should approximate the
    1 right ventricular diastolic pressure.
    2 right atrial pressure.
    3 right ventricular systolic pressure.
    4 pulmonary artery occlusive pressure.

8. Which of the following is used to prevent complications of tension pneumothorax and venous thromboembolism during insertion of a pulmonary artery catheter?
    1 Obtain a chest x-ray before insertion.
    2 Check the patient's partial thromboplastin time.
    3 Place the patient in the Trendelenburg position.
    4 Turn the patient on his or her right side.

9. Which port must be connected to a transducer to allow waveform analysis during insertion of a pulmonary artery catheter?
    1 Pulmonary artery distal
    2 Proximal injectate port
    3 Proximal infusion port
    4 Cardiac output port

10. During the insertion of a pulmonary artery catheter, your patient develops a run of ventricular tachycardia as the catheter passes through the right ventricle. What should you do?
    1 Administer a bolus of 100 mg lidocaine intravenous push.
    2 Nothing. This response is expected.
    3 Cardiovert the patient with 200 joules.
    4 Administer a bolus of 1 mg epinephrine intravenous push.

CHAPTER 7

Pulmonary Artery Pressures and Waveforms

1. Normal pulmonary artery systolic and diastolic pressures are:
   1 120/80 mm Hg.
   2 20/5 mm Hg.
   3 25/15 mm Hg.
   4 45/25 mm Hg.

2. Which scale would be the best to use in a patient with pulmonary hypertension and a pulmonary artery pressure of 56/35 mm Hg?
   1 0–40 mm Hg
   2 0–60 mm Hg
   3 0–200 mm Hg
   4 0–300 mm Hg

3. Which one of the following statements about respiratory variation is *true*?
   1 Pulmonary artery pressure rises during inspiration in a spontaneously breathing patient.
   2 Pulmonary artery pressure falls during inspiration in a mechanically ventilated patient.
   3 Pulmonary artery pressures should be read at peak inspiration.
   4 Pulmonary artery pressures should be read at end-expiration.

4. Left ventricular preload is measured clinically with a pulmonary artery catheter by obtaining a
   1 systemic vascular resistance.
   2 contractility pressure.
   3 pulmonary artery systolic pressure.
   4 pulmonary artery occlusive pressure (PAOP/PCWP).

5. In determining the amount of air used to wedge a pulmonary artery catheter, the best guideline to use is
   1 inflate until the wedge waveform is greater than the systolic.
   2 always instill $1^{1}/_{2}$ cc air.
   3 instill the same amount of air used with the previous wedge.
   4 inflate just until the wedge waveform appears.

6. Which of the following may be ordered to **increase** preload in a hypovolemic patient?
   1 diuretics
   2 volume
   3 vasopressors
   4 vasodilators

Camel comments:

CHAPTER 7—cont'd

7. Which of the following are within normal limits?
   1 PAP 34/24 mm Hg   PAOP 24 mm Hg
   2 PAP 40/20 mm Hg   PAOP 10 mm Hg
   3 PAP 30/20 mm Hg   PAOP 20 mm Hg
   4 PAP 24/14 mm Hg   PAOP 12 mm Hg

8. A pulmonary artery catheter is inserted in a patient with left ventricular failure. While deflating the balloon after wedging, the nurse notes blood in the balloon catheter. Which of the following is the most appropriate action?
   1 Change the syringe to prevent infection.
   2 Check to see whether blood may be aspirated from the site.
   3 Inject 1.5 ml of air to see if wedging is still possible.
   4 Remove the syringe, close it with a dead-end cap and mark "Do not use."

9. A patient develops extreme dyspnea, anxiety, coughing, and expectoration of pink frothy sputum. Heart rate is 120 bpm. Breath sounds reveal inspiratory and expiratory wheezes, rhonchi, and crackles throughout both lung fields. The PAOP is 30 mm Hg. Which of the following is the most likely diagnosis?
   1 Pulmonary embolus
   2 Pneumonia
   3 Pulmonary edema
   4 Cardiogenic shock

10. Preload-reducing drugs either eliminate fluid from the body or cause excess fluid to pool in the venous capacitance beds. Both of these accomplish the goal of decreasing
    1 cardiac output.
    2 afterload.
    3 peripheral vascular resistance.
    4 venous return.

CHAPTER 8

Cardiac Output Measurements & Hemodynamic Calculations

1. Another name for systemic vascular resistance is
   1 preload.
   2 afterload.
   3 contractility.
   4 pulmonary artery diastolic pressure.

2. The afterload pressure is important because it is a measure of
   1 how forcefully the heart contracts.
   2 how much volume the left ventricle has to pump out.
   3 how much resistance the left ventricle has to pump against.
   4 the mean arterial blood pressure.

3. Normal values for systemic vascular resistance are
   1 5 to 6 L/min.
   2 120/80 mm Hg.
   3 800 to 1400 dyne/sec/cm^{-5}.
   4 5 to 15 mm Hg.

4. The afterload pressure for the right ventricle would be the
   1 pulmonary vascular resistance.
   2 systemic vascular resistance.
   3 pulmonary artery occlusive pressure.
   4 pulmonary artery pressure.

5. The formula for obtaining a systemic afterload pressure is
   1 stroke volume multiplied by heart rate.
   2 cardiac output divided by body surface area.
   3 two multiplied by diastolic pressure plus systolic pressure. Divide this total by three.
   4 mean arterial pressure minus central venous pressure and then multiplied by 80. Divide this total by the cardiac output.

6. Normal cardiac output is
   1 2 to 3 L/min.
   2 4 to 8 L/min.
   3 1 to 2 L/min.
   4 10 to 12 L/min.

7. Stroke volume is defined as the difference between the amount of blood in the ventricle at the end of diastole and the amount at the end of systole or the amount pumped out with each beat. The ratio of stroke volume to end-diastolic volume, which is expressed as a percentage, is the
   1 cardiac index.
   2 left ventricular stroke work index.
   3 ejection fraction.
   4 preload.

CHAPTER *8*—cont'd

8. Determinants of stroke volume include all of the following *except*
   1 preload.
   2 afterload.
   3 contractility.
   4 heart rate.

9. Contractility is defined as the
   1 force of contraction.
   2 resistance against which the heart must pump.
   3 volume of the ventricular cavity.
   4 amount of blood pumped with each beat.

10. Which of the following variables is(are) **not** considered in deciding which computation constant to use in computing cardiac output?
   1 Amount of injectate
   2 Temperature of injectate
   3 Type and size of pulmonary catheter
   4 Level of transducer

CHAPTER *9*

Mixed Venous Oxygen Monitoring

1. To monitor mixed venous oxygen levels, which one of the following is needed?
   1 Arterial line
   2 Central venous line
   3 Electrocardiographic monitor
   4 Pulmonary artery catheter

2. Mrs. Johnson is in acute pain, which could result in a(an)
   1 decrease in venous oxygen saturation as a result of increased oxygen consumption.
   2 increase in venous oxygen saturation as a result of increased oxygen consumption.
   3 decrease in venous oxygen saturation as a result of decreased oxygen consumption.
   4 increase in venous oxygen saturation as a result of decreased oxygen consumption.

3. Mixed venous oxygen consumption allows us to measure the
   1 amount of oxygen in arterial blood.
   2 balance between oxygen supply and demand.
   3 balance between carbon dioxide supply and demand.
   4 amount of carbon dioxide in venous blood.

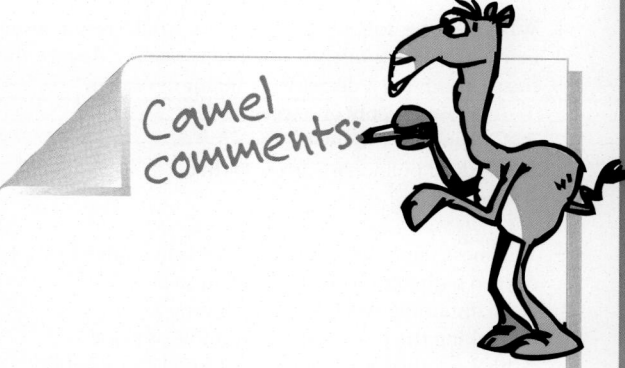
Camel comments:

CHAPTER *9*—cont'd

4. Which of the following conditions would result in an increased venous oxygen saturation reading despite the tissues receiving a decreased amount of oxygen?
   1 Increased supply of oxygen
   2 Cirrhosis of the liver
   3 Wedged pulmonary artery catheter
   4 Sepsis

5. The most important aspect of inserting a mixed venous oxygen catheter for the bedside nurse is
   1 maintaining strict sterile technique.
   2 making the patient as comfortable as possible.
   3 making the physician as comfortable as possible.
   4 observing the pulse oximetry probe for any kind of ectopy.

6. While inserting a pulmonary artery catheter, the balloon on the tip of the catheter should be inflated when the catheter passes into the
   1 vena cava.
   2 right atrium.
   3 right ventricle.
   4 pulmonary artery.

4. In impedance cardiography, the difference between the electrical current introduced and the current sensed is measured in
   1 joules.
   2 ohms.
   3 kilowatts.
   4 milliamperes.

5. The term used for measurement of preload in impedance cardiography is
   1 systemic vascular resistance.
   2 pulmonary artery occlusive pressure.
   3 stroke work index.
   4 thoracic fluid content.

6. Esophageal Doppler monitoring produces a two-dimensional (velocity and time) physiologic waveform that represents pulsatile blood flow in the
   1 coronary arteries.
   2 esophagus.
   3 descending aorta.
   4 ascending aorta.

CHAPTER *10*

Noninvasive Hemodynamic Monitoring

1. Which diagnostic test is considered the gold standard for hemodynamic measurement?
   1 Cardiac catheterization
   2 Impedance cardiography
   3 Pulmonary artery catheterization
   4 Two-dimensional echocardiography

2. Blood is a good conductor of electrical energy. Therefore its impedance is _____.

3. Impedance cardiography is measured noninvasively with four pairs of electrodes. Two pairs are current-emitting electrodes and two pairs serve as
   1 sensing electrodes.
   2 pacing electrodes.
   3 monitoring electrodes.
   4 defibrillation electrodes.

NCLEX® CHAPTER *1* ANSWERS

1.2   Blood returns to the heart via the superior or inferior vena cava, and then blood flows to the right atrium, right ventricle, pulmonary artery, lungs (pulmonary capillary bed), pulmonary veins, left atrium, left ventricle, aorta, and systemic circulation. Forward blood flow does not go from the left ventricle to the pulmonary veins. Blood flows from the right ventricle to the pulmonary artery. Blood flows from the left atrium to the left ventricle.

2.1   Systole is the phase of contraction when blood is being ejected from the ventricles. Diastole is the phase during which the ventricles are filling with blood. Filling and resting occur during diastole.

3.2   Diastole refers to filling the ventricles. Systole refers to the contraction of the ventricles. Contraction and ejection of blood occur during systole.

4.2   The right ventricle pumps blood into the pulmonary artery. The right atrium delivers blood to the right ventricle. The left atrium delivers blood to the left ventricle. The left ventricle pumps blood into the aorta.

5.2   The mitral and tricuspid valves are open during diastole. The pulmonic and aortic valves are closed during diastole. The aortic valve is closed during diastole, and the tricuspid valve is open. The mitral valve is open during diastole, and the pulmonic valve is closed.

6.3   The electrical conduction system is the stimulus for the heart to pump (contract). Filling is the phase of diastole, not contraction. Relaxation is the resting and filling phase of the heart. Diastole is the filling phase; ventricular diastole occurs during the electrical phase of atrioventricular holding.

7.2   The pulmonic valve is open, leaving an open circuit to the aortic valve, which is closed. During diastole the tricuspid valve is open but the pulmonic valve is closed. The aortic valve is closed and the tricuspid valve is open, but the pulmonic valve is also closed, which allows the circuit to be open from the tricuspid valve to the pulmonic valve. A circuit from the pulmonic valve to the aorta also exists. The pulmonic valve is closed, beginning a circuit from the pulmonary artery, through the pulmonary capillary bed to the pulmonary veins, and to the left atrium. However, the circuit does not stop at the mitral valve because it is open; the circuit would continue to the aortic valve.

Camel comments:

NCLEX® CHAPTER *1* ANSWERS—cont'd

8.2 Left ventricular end–diastolic volume is the amount of blood that is in the ventricle just before ejection. Left ventricular end–systolic volume is the amount of blood that remains in the left ventricle at the end of systole. The portion of the volume the left ventricle ejects during diastole (approximately 70% of the total volume at the end of diastole) is referred to as ejection fraction. Stroke volume is the volume of blood that is ejected during systole.

9.2 Respiration is the movement of respiratory gas molecules across the cell. Ventilation is the exchange of oxygen and carbon dioxide between the atmosphere and lungs. Respiration is dependent on distribution of gases between the upper airways and the alveoli. Inhalation is the breathing in of a substance.

10.3 Pulmonary vascular resistance is the pressure the right ventricle must overcome to promote forward flow of blood through the pulmonary circulation. Systemic vascular resistance is the pressure the left ventricle must overcome to eject blood. Distribution refers to flow. Coronary artery circulation is the distribution of blood to the coronary arteries.

NCLEX® CHAPTER *2* ANSWERS

1.3 Contractility is the degree of ventricular stretch. Preload is the volume in the left ventricle at the end of diastole. Afterload is the resistance against which the left ventricle has to work. Cardiac output is the amount of blood ejected from the ventricles in 1 minute.

2.2 The electrical conduction system provides the stimulation for depolarization of cardiac cells, which results in contraction. Venous return to the heart results in right atrial filling. The return from the pulmonary capillary bed via the pulmonary veins results in left atrium filling. Systemic vascular resistance is reflective of afterload. Afterload is the resistance against which the left ventricle works.

3.1 The formula for cardiac output equals stroke volume multiplied by heart rate. The cardiac output formula does not include patient weight. Contractility is one of the parameters that influences stroke volume. Preload and afterload should also be considered. Stroke volume is included in the formula for cardiac output, but contractility is one of the parameters for stroke volume.

4.3 Heart rate is not a parameter of stroke volume. However, it is part of the formula for cardiac output. Preload, afterload, and contractility are parameters of stroke volume.

5.3 Preload is a measurement of left ventricular end–diastolic pressure, which is reflective of left ventricular–end diastolic volume. SVR is reflective of afterload. Contractility is a component of stroke volume. Preload is not the only parameter considered in cardiac output.

6.4 Afterload is the resistance against which the left ventricle works. It is measured by obtaining systemic vascular resistance. Pulmonary capillary wedge pressure is reflective of preload. Cardiac output considers stroke volume and heart rate. Contractility is one component of stroke volume.

7.2 Inotropic means affecting contractility. Chronotropic refers to affecting rate. Vasoactive means affecting the blood vessels. Vasodilatory means causing dilation of the vessels.

8.2 A pulmonary capillary wedge pressure or PAOP is reflective of left ventricular–end diastolic volume pressure or preload. Systemic vascular resistance is reflective of afterload. Left ventricular stroke work index is reflective of contractility. Pulmonary artery systolic pressure reflects pressure in the pulmonary artery during systole when the mitral valve is closed, thus only reflecting left atrial pressure.

9.2 Systemic vascular resistance is a reflection of the peripheral resistance during mean aortic pressure. Pulmonary venous resistances reflects the resistance against which the right ventricle works (the resistance from the lungs). Mean arterial pressure is a reflection of the perfusion pressure to vital organs. Pulmonary capillary wedge pressure reflects left ventricular–end diastolic pressure.

10.3 Hypoxia, myocardial scar tissue, and parasympathetic stimulation decrease contractility. Miscellaneous influences that decrease myocardial contractility include hypoxia, hyperkalemia, hypercarbia, hyponatremia, and myocardial scar tissue. Sympathetic stimulation increases contractility.

NCLEX® CHAPTER *3* ANSWERS

1.3 A pulmonary artery catheter can measure pulmonary artery systolic, diastolic, and central venous pressures. A separate catheter must be inserted in an artery to measure arterial pressures.

2.4 Potential complications of pulmonary artery pressure monitoring include ventricular irritability and ectopy, heart blocks, pulmonary artery rupture, and potential for emboli.

NCLEX® CHAPTER *3* ANSWERS—cont'd

3.4 The Allen's test is used to detect appropriate collateral circulation in the ulnar artery. A 12-lead electrocardiogram is used to detect ischemia in the heart. A complete blood count is used to determine hemoglobin, hematocrit, and blood cell counts. A mixed venous blood gas is used to detect oxygen consumption.

4.1 Transducers used in hemodynamic monitoring should be leveled to the phlebostatic axis because the right atrium is the level that references heart pressures. The position of the left lower lung is too low. The right hand position can be variable (too low or too high) and would be inaccurate. The position of the right internal jugular vein is too high and would be inaccurate.

5.3 When zeroing a transducer, the stopcock is open to the air and closed to the patient. The stopcock should be open to the air and closed to the patient to allow the transducer to have an air reference.

6.4 The square wave test is used to test the ability of the fluid-filled monitoring system to reproduce accurately the patient's pressure on the monitor. The Allen's test is used to detect appropriate collateral circulation in the ulnar artery. The Schilling test is a vitamin B_{12}–absorption test. Ice water calorics test for brainstem integrity in the comatose patient.

7.2 The phlebostatic axis is located at the fourth intercostal space, midaxillary line. The second intercostal space, midclavicular position is referred to as the pulmonic area for listening to heart sounds. The level of the fifth intercostal space, anterior axillary position is the position of the V5 recording electrode on a 12-lead electrocardiogram. The fifth intercostal space, lower left sternal border can be used when listening for heart sounds.

8.4 To obtain reliable hemodynamic measurements, the nurse should complete all of the following: level and zero the transducer, ensure proper patient positioning, and ensure the system is fluid filled, air-bubble free, and that all connections are tightened.

9.1 The pressure bag on the flush solution should be inflated to 300 mm Hg. An inflation of 200 mm Hg or 250 mm Hg is insufficient pressure to maintain a flush of 3 ml per hour. An inflation of 350 mm Hg exceeds the recommended amount of pressure.

10.2 Patient preparation for hemodynamic monitoring includes all of the following: washing hands, having emergency equipment readily available, explaining the procedure to the patient, and ensuring consent forms are signed.

Camel comments:

NCLEX® CHAPTER 4 ANSWERS

1.3 Arterial pressure monitoring lines are used only as an invasive, direct way to monitor blood pressure and to obtain frequent blood samples. Arterial lines are not used to administer medications because of the high risk of thrombosis to the affected extremity. An arterial line is used to directly measure a continuous blood pressure in a patient receiving an intravenous vasoactive medication that requires titrating. A patient who has a systolic blood pressure less than 85 mm Hg would be considered hemodynamically unstable; arterial pressure monitoring would be the preferred method for measuing and monitoring blood pressure. The patient requiring frequent blood sampling would benefit from an arterial line because the blood samples could be obtained from the line, not from a direct needle stick.

2.1 The Allen's test is performed to determine ulnar artery patency. Chvostek's test is performed by tapping on the facial nerve to elicit an abnormal facial muscle spasm to determine the degree of hypocalcemia. Homan's test is performed by dorsiflexing the foot to elicit pain in the calf to indicate possible thrombophlebitis or thrombosis. Trousseau's test is performed by inflating a blood pressure cuff to elicit a carpal spasm to determine the presence of latent tetany.

3.3 A pedal artery insertion is primarily chosen because other arterial insertion sites are not available. The patient will not be able to walk or stand with a pedal arterial line because the site will need to be immobilized. In addition, the patient is at great risk for developing a thrombotic occlusion, and the waveform is predisposed to artifact and erroneous readings.

4.1 An overdamped waveform is characterized by a smooth waveform that loses its landmarks. Air bubbles in the system is one cause of an overdamped waveform; another cause is an empty flush bag. Immobilization would result in greater accuracy of the reading and would not cause overdamping or underdamping. A patient's febrile state would have a tendency to cause underdamping, not overdamping.

5.4 It is important that the circulation status of the extremity in which the arterial catheter is placed is assessed on an ongoing basis. Assessing the patient's heart sounds, level of consciousness, bilateral pupil responses, or ability to move and feel the opposite (left) foot is not directly related to the presence of a right femoral arterial line.

6.2 The dicrotic notch depicts the closure of the aortic valve. The dicrotic notch has notch has nothing to do with the tricuspid, pulmonic, or mitral valves

7.3 Increased blood flow to the extremity is not a complication of arterial line placement. A decreased distal blood flow to the extremity involved would be a complication of an arterial line because the catheter could cause a slight or complete occlusion. An infection, air embolism, and exsanguinations or hemorrhage are all possible complications that may occur from the placement of an arterial line.

8.4 Direct, firm pressure must be applied to the site for 5 to 10 minutes after the arterial catheter has been removed.

9.1 An underdamped waveform is characterized by an exaggeration of systolic pressure and may be caused by an excessive tubing length greater than 3 to 4 feet. Numerous or additional stopcocks, bent or kinked tubing, and an empty flush bag can cause overdamping.

10.4 Pressure is released on the ulnar artery during the performance of the Allen's test to determine whether blood is adequately flowing into the hand. The axillary and brachial arteries are not used in the performance of the Allen's test. The radial artery is used in the performance of the Allen's test but remains occluded when the Allen's test is performed.

NCLEX® CHAPTER 5 ANSWERS

1.2 Although central venous pressure correlates with left heart pressure in patients with normal heart and lungs, it most directly correlates to right atrial pressure.

2.3 The normal central venous pressure ranges from 0 to 8 mm Hg. Central venous pressure ranges from 8 to 19 mm Hg; a range of 6 to 12 mm Hg is too high and would indicate volume overload or right heart failure. A central venous pressure range of 0 to 4 mm Hg is too low and may indicate a volume deficit or hypovolemia.

3.1 The circulation nurse is directly responsible for monitoring central venous catheter insertion and for providing emotional support to the patient. The nurse who is scrubbed and assisting with the procedure would be responsible for gathering equipment, assisting the physician, and watching the monitor.

NCLEX® CHAPTER 5 ANSWERS—cont'd

4.3 If the patient's clinical condition allows, the patient should be placed flat and supine for a central venous pressure reading. Trendelenburg and left side positions would provide an inaccurate reading. If the patient is orthopneic, the central venous pressure may be read with the head of the bed elevated; however, this position is not ideal.

5.4 The phlebostatic axis, fourth intercostal space, midaxillary line, is the correct place to measure central venous pressure. The midaxillary line is not a complete answer. A measurement at the intramammary line or the left ventricle would provide a false reading.

6.1 The central venous pressure is measured at the end of expiration. Central venous pressure should not be measured at the beginning or end of inspiration because inspiration raises the intrathoracic pressure and may increase central venous pressure.

7.2 A low central venous pressure may indicate hypovolemia. Fluid overload, left heart failure, and cardiac tamponade would cause an elevated central venous pressure.

8.4 The response of the central venous pressure to a fluid challenge will help determine the patient's fluid status (whether the patient is hypovolemic). Continuous readings provide a trend but are not responses to a specific treatment. Measuring the central venous pressure with the patient on a ventilator is appropriate if the patient is mechanically ventilated, but it alone will not help determine whether the patient is hypovolemic. Reading the central venous pressure with the patient in different positions will produce a number of false readings. The central venous pressure should always be measured with the patient in the same position.

9.2 Although infection, hemorrhage, and pneumothorax are serious complications, air embolus can cause the most rapid cardiovascular collapse and is therefore the most immediate life-threatening complication related to central venous catheters.

10.1 There should be minimal resistance when removing a central venous catheter. If some resistance is felt, this resistance indicates a possible problem that should be investigated before proceeding with the removal of the central venous catheter.

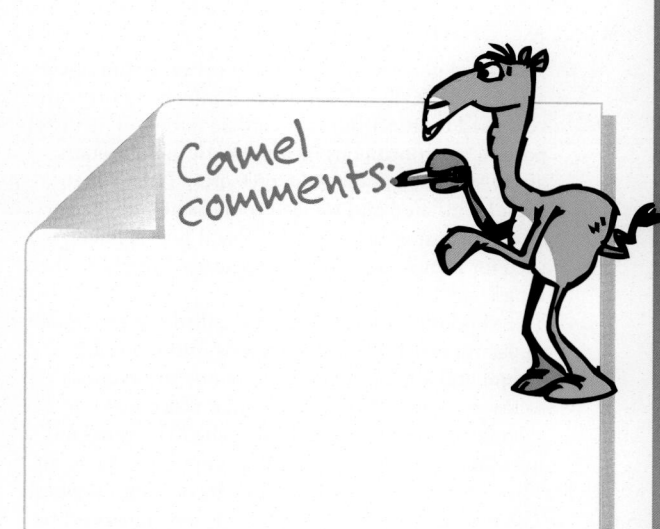

Camel comments:

NCLEX® CHAPTER *6* ANSWERS

1.1 The distal port is connected to a pressure transducer and a flush device. The proximal injectate port is the port used to inject fluid for cardiac output. The distal port allows continuous measurement of pulmonary artery systolic and diastolic pressures. The balloon must be inflated and wedged to measure pulmonary artery occlusion pressure. The distal port is never used for intravenous infusion; it leads directly to the lungs.

2.4 The venous infusion port is also called the proximal infusion port. This lumen empties into the right atrium and allows the infusion of any intravenous solution or drug. Systemic vascular resistance is a calculated—not measured—pressure. The proximal injectate port is used for cardiac output measurement. The distal lumen is used to draw mixed venous gases.

3.1 The full amount or $1^1/_2$ ml of air is recommended to prevent trauma to the cardiac vessels, chambers, and valves during insertion. Either $^1/_2$ ml or 1 ml of air would not sufficiently inflate the balloons. Two milliliters of air would overinflate and possibly burst the balloon.

4.2 Preload, afterload, and contractility are the three parameters of stroke volume. Cardiac output equals stroke volume times heart rate. Excitability, conductivity, and automaticity relate to the heart's conduction system. Heart rate is a determinate of cardiac output, not stroke volume. Preload, afterload, and contractility affect blood pressure.

5.4 The dicrotic notch on the PA waveform is caused by the closure of the pulmonic valve. It represents the onset of diastole. The initial brisk upstroke of the arterial waveform represents the opening of the aortic valve. The dicrotic notch on an arterial waveform represents closure of the aortic valve and the onset of diastole. The pulmonary waveform represents the opening of the pulmonic valve.

6.2 The transducer must be leveled at the fourth intercostal space, midaxillary line or the patient's right atrium. An imaginary line should be drawn between this level and the side port of the transducer (the air-fluid interface). If the transducer is too high, then the readings will be erroneously low. If the transducer is too low, then the readings will be erroneously high. The pressure cuff on the solution bag should be maintained at 300 mm Hg. The monitor should be set on a scale of 0 to 40 mm Hg. Vented caps should be replaced with nonvented caps on all stopcock ports after flushing.

7.3 The pulmonic valve is open during systole. Therefore the pressures between the two chambers on either side of the valve will equilibrate during systole. However, during diastole, the pulmonic valve closes and the pulmonary artery and right ventricle pressures will be different. The right ventricle diastolic pressure reflects the tone of the right ventricle when it is filling from the right atrium and not pumping. The pulmonary artery diastolic pressure will be higher because the pulmonic valve closes during diastole, and pressure is reflected back from the pulmonary vasculature. The right atrium pressure is a mean pressure, which is not related to the pulmonary artery systolic pressure. The pulmonary artery occlusion pressure is determined by wedging the catheter and is not affected by the pulmonary artery systolic pressure.

8.3 Placing the patient in the Trendelenburg position engorges the subclavian vessels and increases the central venous pressure. This position makes the vessels more prominent and therefore decreases the chance of inadvertent puncture of a lung. A chest x-ray is obtained after the procedure to verify placement and to rule out a pneumothorax. The partial thromboplastin time would be related to bleeding complications. No benefit exists in turning the patient to his or her right side.

9.1 The pulmonary artery distal port must be connected to the transducer because it is the port that guides the catheter tip as it floats through the heart and blood vessels. The proximal injectate port, proximal infusion port, and cardiac output port can all be connected after initial insertion. The proximal injectate port is connected to a transducer port. The proximal infusion port can be connected to any intravenous solution. The cardiac output port is connected to a Y-connector cable with one end to the monitor and one end to the thermoset used for measuring the carbon dioxide level.

10.2 Ventricular irritability may occur as the tip of the catheter passes through the right ventricle. This response is mechanical in nature and should resolve once the catheter passes into the pulmonary artery. Lidocaine is usually not necessary. Cardioversion would not be indicated unless the ventricular tachycardia is sustained and the patient becomes hemodynamically unstable. Epinephrine is inappropriate; it would aggravate the ventricular tachycardia.

NCLEX® CHAPTER 7 ANSWERS

1.3 Pulmonary artery pressures are considerably lower than arterial pressures. A normal pulmonary artery systolic pressure is 25 mm Hg; 15 mm Hg is a normal pulmonary artery diastolic pressure; therefore 25/15 is a normal pulmonary artery pressure measurement. A normal systemic arterial pressure is 120/80 mm Hg. A normal right ventricular pressure is 20/5 mm Hg. Elevated pulmonary artery systolic and diastolic pressures would be reflected by 45/25 mm Hg.

2.2 A scale of 0 to 60 mm Hg would allow the entire waveform to appear on the oscilloscope screen. A smaller scale would cut off the waveform. A scale of 0 to 40 mm Hg is used for normal pulmonary artery pressures, but a systolic pressure of 56 mm Hg will go off the top of this scale. A larger scale (0 to 200 mm Hg or 0 to 300 mm Hg) would cause the waveform to appear too small to read.

3.4 Regardless of whether the patient is spontaneously breathing or on a ventilator, pulmonary artery pressures should be obtained at end-expiration when minimal interference occurs with respiration. Pulmonary artery pressure falls with inspiration in a spontaneously breathing patient. The measurement should therefore be taken at the highest point before the decrease (or end-expiration). Pulmonary artery pressures rise with inspiration on a mechanically ventilated patient. The measurement should therefore be taken at the lowest point before the increase (or end-expiration). All measurements should be taken at end-expiration while the chest is quiet— not on inspiration when the dynamics of movement would increase the respiratory artifact.

4.4 By wedging the catheter in a pulmonary arteriole, back pressure from the left side of the heart is measured. The pulmonary artery occlusion pressure is an indirect measurement of the left atrial and left ventricular end–diastolic pressures, which are the preload for the left ventricle. Systemic vascular resistance measures afterload. Contractility is measured by left ventricular stroke work index. Pulmonary artery systolic pressure reflects pulmonary or right-sided pressures.

5.4 The tip of the catheter can float, and the position may be slightly different each time the catheter is wedged. In addition, the blood vessels may be more vasodilated or vasoconstricted because of hemodynamic changes. Therefore the balloon volume may differ each time the catheter is wedged. Regardless of how much air is needed to wedge the catheter, the goal is to inflate the balloon slowly, just until the wedge waveform appears. This precaution will

Camel comments:

NCLEX® CHAPTER 7 ANSWERS—cont'd

prevent overwedging and balloon rupture. The wedge waveform should never be greater than the systolic; it should be equal to or less than the diastolic. Although $1^1/2$ ml is the maximum amount of air that the syringe will hold, the entire amount may not be needed to inflate the balloon. The distal tip could have migrated and may take more or less air than the previous wedge.

6.2   Patients with hypovolemia will have decreased preload; volume is needed. Diuretics would aggravate the problem of hypovolemia. Vasopressors are only indicated when volume is ineffective. Vasodilators would aggravate the problem by causing an increase in the relative hypovolemia.

7.4   These measurements (PAP, 24/14 mm Hg; PAOP, 12 mm Hg) most closely reflect normal pulmonary artery pressures. Normal pulmonary artery systolic pressure is 20 to 33 mm Hg. Normal pulmonary artery diastolic pressure is 10 to 15 mm Hg. Normal pulmonary artery occlusion pressure is 4 to 12 mm Hg. Pulmonary artery pressures of 34/24 mm Hg and pulmonary artery occlusion pressure of 24 mm Hg are higher than normal. Pulmonary artery pressures of 40/20 mm Hg and pulmonary artery occlusion pressure of 10 mm Hg are incorrect because the pulmonary artery pressures are high even though the wedge is normal. Pulmonary artery pressures of 30/20 mm Hg and pulmonary artery occlusion pressure of 20 mm Hg is incorrect because the pulmonary artery occlusion pressure is high even though the pulmonary artery pressures are normal.

8.4   Blood in the syringe suggests that the balloon has ruptured. The balloon port should no longer be used. Infection control is not the primary issue in this case. Checking to see whether blood may be aspirated from the site is unnecessary. If the balloon is ruptured, injecting air could cause an air embolus, causing the air to go directly into circulation.

9.3   Pink, frothy, sputum, crackles on auscultation, dyspnea, and an elevated wedge pressure are all signs of pulmonary edema. These symptoms would not be present in pulmonary embolus or cardiogenic shock.

10.4   Venous return is the main determinant of preload. Diuretics and venous vasodilators both decrease venous return and therefore preload. Cardiac output may be indirectly influenced by preload; however, cardiac output is not the best answer. Afterload is another name for peripheral vascular resistance and is more influenced by arteriolar tone rather than by volume.

NCLEX® CHAPTER 8 ANSWERS

1.2   Left ventricle afterload is synonymous with systemic vascular resistance. It is the resistance against which the left ventricle must pump during systole. The arteries that are receiving the blood during systole come "after" the heart. Preload deals with volume, not resistance. Contractility deals with the force of the cardiac contraction. Pulmonary, not systemic, resistance mainly determines diastolic pressure.

2.3   The afterload pressure is important because it is a measure of how much resistance against which the left ventricle has to pump. This pressure is important because it reflects the status of the arterioles (whether they are constricted or dilated), thereby helping to determine proper treatment. How forcefully the heart contracts is the definition of contractility. Preload is how much volume the left ventricle has to pump out. The mean arterial pressure is just one factor in calculating afterload.

3.3   Systemic vascular resistance is not a pressure measurement but a resistance measurement. It is measured in $dynes/sec/cm^{-5}$. A normal range is 800 to 1400 $dynes/sec/cm^{-5}$. Average cardiac output is 5 to 6 L/min. Average blood pressure is 120/80 mm Hg. Afterload is not measured in mm Hg, therefore 5 to 15 mm Hg is incorrect.

4.1   The resistance in the pulmonary arterioles, which comes "after" the right ventricle and receives the blood ejected during systole, determines the afterload for the right ventricle. Systemic vascular resistance measures peripheral resistance. Pulmonary artery occlusion pressure measures left ventricular preload. Pulmonary artery pressure has systolic and diastolic components.

5.4   The mathematical formula for measuring afterload is the following: the mean arterial pressure, minus the central venous pressure; this answer is then divided by cardiac output; this quotient is then multiplied by 80. It is determined by factors affecting peripheral resistance. Cardiac output equals stroke volume multiplied by heart rate. The formula for cardiac index is cardiac output divided by body surface area. The formula for mean arterial pressure is 2 multiplied by diastolic pressure plus systolic pressure; this answer is then divided by 3.

NCLEX® CHAPTER *8* ANSWERS—cont'd

6.2   Cardiac output is the amount of blood pumped out of the heart per minute. The stroke volume times the heart rate determines cardiac output. Normal stroke volume is approximately 70 ml. Normal heart rate is approximately 70 beats per minute. Therefore normal cardiac output equals 4 to 8 L/min. Four liters would be normal for a small person. Eight liters would be normal for a large person. Between 2 and 3 L/min or 1 to 2 L/min would be diminished cardiac outputs. Between 10 and 12 L/min would be an elevated cardiac output.

7.3   Ejection fraction is the number (percentage) often used to quantify left ventricular function. It can be invasively measured by catheter or noninvasively by echocardiogram. The cardiac index equals cardiac output corrected for body size. Left ventricular stroke work index is a measure of left ventricular contractility. Preload is the volume of blood remaining in the left ventricle at the end of diastole.

8.4   Heart rate is not a major determinant in stroke volume, although it IS a factor in cardiac output. The determinants of stroke volume are preload, afterload, and contractility.

9.1   Contractility is defined as the force of left ventricular contraction or how hard the heart squeezes to pump out the blood during systole. The resistance against which the heart must pump is a measure of afterload. The volume of ventricular cavity is a measure of preload. The amount of blood pumped with each beat is the definition of stroke volume.

10.4 The level of the transducer, although important in determining accurate pressure measurements, is not a factor in choosing a computation constant. The amount of injectate, temperature of the injectate, and type and size of the pulmonary artery catheter are all factors in determining a computation constant.

NCLEX® CHAPTER *9* ANSWERS

1.4   Mixed venous oxygen saturation monitoring is a complex process, requiring a significant amount of time and material. It is important that the nurse not confuse this type of monitoring with arterial saturation or pulse oximetry monitoring. An arterial line would monitor arterial blood pressure. A central venous line would monitor the amount of pressure at the right atrium of the heart, an indirect measure of the amount of fluid in the circulation. An electrocardiogram would monitor the electrical rhythm of the impulses that pass through the heart.

Camel comments:

NCLEX® CHAPTER *9* ANSWERS—cont'd

2.1 Pain results from stimulation of the sympathetic nervous system, which causes a drop in venous oxygen saturation and increased oxygen consumption. It is important for the nurse to realize that patients who are in pain have real physiologic changes and that these changes may result in increased consumption of oxygen. This increased consumption can be dangerous for patients who are severely ill or have decreased cardiac reserves. Increased oxygen consumption ordinarily increases venous oxygen saturation. Pain increases respiratory rate and sympathetic nervous system stimulation, thereby increasing oxygen consumption.

3.2 Mixed venous oxygen consumption allows the measurement of the balance between oxygen supply and demand. Understanding the purpose of monitoring mixed venous oxygen saturation alerts the nurse to its importance and provides cues for other aspects of the patient's condition that could have an affect on this information. Oxygen and carbon dioxide levels in arterial blood can be measured far more easily by obtaining an arterial blood gas reading. Carbon dioxide supply and demand is very difficult to measure; it usually involves a complex process called calorimetry.

4.4 Sepsis would result in an increased venous oxygen saturation reading despite tissues receiving a decreased amount of oxygen. There are exceptions to every rule, and sepsis is one of these exceptions. Despite the high level of oxygen consumption, the low circulating blood pressure results in inadequate circulation to the body, thus "trapping" the oxygen stores in the core. An increased oxygen supply may increase this reading, but ordinarily, increased oxygen will also increase tissue oxygenation. Although end-stage liver disease may have an effect on venous oxygen saturation, cirrhosis does not ordinarily result in such acute changes in venous oxygen saturation. A wedged pulmonary artery catheter provides isolated left heart measurements and does not affect venous oxygen saturation.

5.1 The most important aspect of inserting a mixed venous oxygen catheter at the bedside is for the nurse to maintain strict sterile technique. The vast majority of hospital acquired complications comes from human error. An archetypical human error in the hospital is a break in aseptic technique. The resulting nosocomial infections result in huge expenditures by hospitals and costs to the patient. It is important to impress on the nurse the importance of vigilance in aseptic technique. Although patient comfort is important, such pursuit should never result in a degradation of sterile technique. Comfort is important but not the most important aspect. The physician's comfort is immaterial to the procedure, except when such discomfort precludes successful catheter insertion. Even then, physician comfort is secondary to sterility. The pulse oximeter probe is a poor monitor for ectopy with numerous false-positive waveforms.

6.2 If the balloon is inflated at the wrong time during the insertion of a pulmonary artery catheter, damage to the patient's heart or valves may result. The balloon must be inflated as the catheter passes into the right atrium. The catheter passes through the vena cava, but inflation of the balloon at this point will not aid in the insertion of the catheter. Inflating the balloon while it passes into the right ventricle makes passage through the right atrium to this point far more difficult. Inflating the balloon as it passes into the pulmonary artery is performed solely for purposes of monitoring, not placement.

NCLEX® CHAPTER *10* ANSWERS

1.3 Pulmonary artery catheterization is the "gold standard" for hemodynamic measurement because it allows for direct pressure measurements. Cardiac catheterization allows for direct pressure measurement, but it is not practical to use at the patient's bedside. Although impedance cardiography is showing promise as a noninvasive tool and correlated well with pulmonary artery catheterization, it is still not the procedure of choice in most cases. Two-dimensional echocardiography can detect many hemodynamic parameters, but it, too, is not the procedure of choice.

2. Blood is a good conductor of electrical energy. Therefore it has low impedance.

3.1 The current is introduced via two pairs of electrodes and sensed by the other two pairs, which will register any drop in voltage. Pacing and defibrillation are not functions of impedance cardiography. Although these two pairs serve to monitor the voltage, this is not the best answer for the posed question.

4.2 In impedance cardiography, the difference between the electrical current introduced and the current sensed is measured in ohms, a measure of resistance. Joules are used to measure defibrillation current. Kilowatts are not used to measure bioelectrical energy. Pacemaker technology uses milliamperes.

NCLEX® CHAPTER *10* ANSWERS—cont'd

5.4 The term used for measurement of preload in impedance cardiography is thoracic fluid content. Greater amounts of fluid reduce impedance; a reduced impedance would correlate with an elevated pulmonary artery occlusion pressure and would suggest volume overload. Systemic vascular resistance is a measure of afterload. Pulmonary artery occlusive pressure is used to measure preload with pulmonary artery catheterization; however, it is not the method used with noninvasive hemodynamic monitoring. The stroke work index is a measure of contractility.

6.3 The physiologic waveform produced in esophageal Doppler monitoring represents pulsatile blood flow in the descending aorta because the probe is directly located adjacent to it. The coronary arteries are not adjacent to the esophagus. Although the transducer probe that emits the sound waves is located in the esophagus, it detects blood flow in the aorta. The ascending aorta is not used because it is too short to be accurate. Further, it is not directly adjacent to the esophagus, and blood flow is too turbulent.

Camel comments:

Index

Printed in the United States
By Bookmasters